THE
DIABETES
BOOK

CHET GALASKA

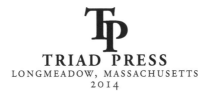

TRIAD PRESS
LONGMEADOW, MASSACHUSETTS
2014

The Diabetes Book

by Chet Galaska

Copyright © 2014 by C.W. Galaska

ISBN: 978-0-9816767-5-3

Library of Congress Control Number: 2014934574

Previously published as *Living on a Tightrope: Coping with Diabetes*

Printed in the U.S.A.

www.thediabetesbook.net

This book is dedicated to

My wife, Lisa
My sons, Jon & Drew
My mom, Virginia
and
My brother Don,
who has provided the kind of support only
someone who has walked in your shoes can offer.

Table of Contents

Acknowledgments

Thanks to everyone who contributed advice and help in writing this book. Deb Ciosek and Laura Maloney-Hastillo were generous in sharing their compelling personal stories.

Christopher R. Kerouac, M.D., and Stephanie M. Hastings, B.A., Coordinator of the 50-Year Medalist Program at the Joslin Diabetes Center, provided valuable insights and comments.

Kelly Henry, R.N., C.D.E., C.P.T. was especially helpful in sharing her extensive hands-on experience with and knowledge of both types of diabetes. Kelly reviewed the text, offered improvements and sent me in directions I wouldn't have gone otherwise. I'm grateful for her help in this project and the dedication she has to her patients.

An Important Note to Readers

This book is for everyone – diabetic or not – who wants a basic understanding of diabetes and some insights into the day to day issues involved in it. People with diabetes and those close to them will probably learn some new things. I know I did in doing the research.

Everyone else can benefit too. The book is written like it's directed toward diabetics but it can help others by throwing light on a threat that's often feared as a dark, mysterious monster lurking around the corner. Once non-diabetics learn of the strides made in treatment and understand diabetes can be treated, they'll discover that the horror shows they imagine do not need to happen. And once they know the symptoms they may more readily seek treatment for themselves or suggest it for others. If people with symptoms get medical help sooner rather than later they'll take a huge step toward staying healthy.

I was in Chicago the week Ron Santo was inducted into the Baseball Hall of Fame. Previously unknown to me, Santo had Type 1 diabetes in the late 1950's and kept it to himself for fear of losing his job. *The Chicago Tribune* ran stories about his battle that I, as a person with diabetes, could relate to. But I realized most people couldn't understand them because they don't know enough about diabetes to appreciate Santo's situation. That's where the idea for this book came from.

Over the next few months I spoke to people about Santo's story and found there's a much greater lack of knowledge about diabetes than I ever dreamed. And it's almost as prevalent among diabetics as it is in the general public. To make matters worse, misinformation and old wives' tales throw monkey wrenches into understanding the realities. Good, caring people often "know" things that simply aren't true and harbor misconceptions that can be counterproductive.

Diabetes is a serious, life-threatening disease that's reached epidemic proportions and the chances are everyone either has it or knows someone who does. Given its prevalence everyone should have a basic knowledge of it.

The Diabetes Book offers this. The information presented is accurate, but please understand it's a general overview and shouldn't be used for medical advice. It simply aims to convey how the two major types of diabetes work, drive home the importance of the patient's active participation in his/her own care and offer some practical advice for living with it. Readers must remember that diabetes affects individuals differently and professionals are needed to develop personal treatment strategies. If the book raises questions—and I hope it does—you should see your medical professional for answers. Believe me, it's a complicated disease and you won't figure it out on your own.

This book isn't comprehensive and I readily acknowledge that many things have been simplified or omitted. For example, the chapter on "Incorrect Common 'Knowledge'" notes that diabetics don't need special foods aside from the normal, healthy diets that are good for everyone. That's true for the vast majority of us but there are exceptions. If you have diabetic kidney disease you'll need a low-protein diet. Or you may have a gluten intolerance possibly caused by the autoimmune system in Type 1's.

My purpose is to help people easily learn about diabetes. If I tried to explain all the "ifs," "ands," "whys" and "buts" it would have become too long, boring and time consuming for most people to read. That would have defeated its purpose, which is to inform as many people as possible.

If you're diabetic you'll need to refine, modify and add to this information as you learn what works in your individual case. If you're not, you'll better understand how it works and have a real idea of what your diabetic friends and relatives are dealing with. I sincerely hope *The Diabetes Book* makes everyone more knowledgeable, curious and committed to good health.

Introduction

When you're diagnosed with diabetes you instantly become a tightrope walker, even if you've got bad balance and a fear of heights. Your constant lifelong task becomes maintaining a blood sugar level as close to normal as possible without going too high or too low. Like every other tightrope walker you need to pay attention and make continual adjustments to stay in balance.

I was diagnosed with Type 1 over 30 years ago and have taken insulin ever since. I'm not a medical professional; I'm just a guy who's had diabetes for a long time and can write plainly about dealing with it day-to-day.

On one hand, diabetes is much harder to control than most non-diabetics imagine. On the other hand, it is manageable and if it's done well diabetics can lead close to normal lives. Both Type 1 and Type 2 diabetes are complex diseases with issues and therapies that vary from person to person. It's been said that because of the complexity of diabetes it's possible no two cases are exactly alike.

Let me tell you my story. I almost never became ill (in fact, I still rarely do) but in the spring of 1981 I got sicker than I can ever remember. I was weak with no appetite and spent a couple of days lying on the sofa reading *The Island* by Peter Benchley. I felt better afterward but over time found I had a lack of energy and developed a constant thirst.

Some time later I was on a business trip and got really thirsty so I drank orange juice to quench it. The high sugar content blasted my blood glucose level through the roof. I became so parched and groggy it was difficult to speak, which made for a difficult sales call. I didn't know what was happening, but it was obvious something was wrong. A few weeks later I went to the Blue Cross/Blue Shield office on business and spotted some pamphlets in the waiting room that described various common medical conditions. I randomly picked one up to kill time and discovered I had all the symptoms it described except for the ones that applied to women. It seemed pretty clear I had diabetes.

I made an appointment with an internist. Our conversation went like this:

"What brings you here?"

"I think I've got diabetes."

He gave me the look he probably gives every hypochrondriac who comes in with their own diagnosis, and then he took a blood sample. He returned and said, "You've got diabetes."

"Can it be treated with pills?" I asked.

"No, you'll need injections."

Even though I wasn't surprised, the official diagnosis still hit me between the eyes. One of my brothers had diabetes and I was aware of some of the difficulties in managing it. I knew my life had changed—but I also knew it wasn't over.

Type 1 and Type 2 diabetes—which are very different—will both be discussed in this book. Some elements of control apply to both types but others are relevant to just one or the other. Regardless of which type you have it'll be helpful to read about both. At the very least, you'll learn what the differences are and be better able to explain your condition to others.

With either type, living with diabetes truly is a question of balance. It requires continual thinking about what you're doing throughout the day and how it will affect your blood glucose level (BGL). And you need to know how to make adjustments to keep your BGL as close to the normal range as possible.

We diabetics have been shanghaied into an adventure we didn't sign up for. But since we're in it we've got to make the most of it. And you know what? You can still have a great life! But you've got to take this seriously and pay attention.

It's important—losing your BGL balance can be as serious as a tightrope walker falling off the wire.

Chapter 1
A Brief History

Diabetes has been diagnosed for thousands of years but effective treatment wasn't available until the early 20th century. To help explain what earlier physicians saw and thought, it's helpful to know how the disease operates.

Diabetes disables the body's ability to metabolize sugar. Excess sugar builds up in the bloodstream, causing the body to try to eliminate it through excessive urination. The medical term is diabetes mellitus, diabetes meaning "excessive urination" and mellitis meaning "honeysweet." It refers to the sweetness of urine containing excessive amounts of sugar expelled by the body.

The ancients recognized there were two types. The first affected younger people who died from it quickly. This would eventually be called "Juvenile Diabetes" but it's also been found to strike adults and is now typically referred to as "Type 1." The second was associated with overweight and sedentary older people who could live for years while enduring debilitating complications. It came to be called "Adult Onset Diabetes" but is now referred to as "Type 2." Both types were always fatal.

The ancient Egyptians noted the frequent urination problem, while their Hindu contemporaries wrote of ants being attracted to the urine of people suffering emaciation. The Greeks thought the disease melted flesh and expelled it. In what has to be one of the worst medical jobs ever, diabetes was diagnosed by "water tasters" who sampled the urine of those suspected of having the disease to detect sweetness. They did this to separate those with a known incurable deadly disease (diabetes) from those who had something else and might be helped.

Over the years therapies included a high fat and protein diet (which was on the right track, because it reduced the amount of sugar-producing starches), eating excessive amounts of sugar (wrong track), an "oat cure" where the patient would eat 8 ounces of butter mixed with 8 ounces of oatmeal every two hours, opium, or a whiskey/black coffee cocktail every two hours. Some were moderately successful in helping temper the symptoms by restricting food consumption and reducing the amount of sugar in the bloodstream, but undereating could cause death by starvation.

Nothing worked. Sometimes the symptoms got temporarily better and other times they got devastatingly worse, but it remained an incurable fatal illness no matter what was tried.

Then in 1889 scientists researching digestion removed the pancreas from a dog. The animal became diabetic, and a huge clue was uncovered. The pancreas—and not the kidneys, as some had speculated—was the source of whatever controlled blood sugar. Dr. Georg Zuelzer extracted the substance from calf pancreases, called it "Acomatrol" and injected it into a comatose diabetic patient. The patient rallied but died when the small supply of what would later be called insulin ran out. This showed that insulin did, in fact, lower blood sugar. But problems cropped up in later experiments, like painful abscesses, fevers and the mysterious, scary symptoms of insulin reactions (more about this later in the book).

With research continuing, the name "insulin" was suggested for the curative pancreatic substance. Insulin means "island" and refers to the "Islets of Langerhans" which had been discovered by Paul Langerhans 40 years earlier. They were enclosed in a fibrous capsule that separated them from the rest of the pancreatic tissue, so they really are islands within the organ. The islets turned out to be home to the beta cells that produced the magic hormone.

In 1920 Frederick Banting, a Canadian medical doctor who suspected that earlier insulin extracts were compromised by enzymes during removal, started his work. Two years later, Banting's purer insulin was injected into a 14 year-old boy. The test was successful and within the year the University of Toronto contracted with Eli Lilly & Co. to mass produce insulin. After thousands of frustrating years, an effective treatment for diabetes was finally available.

Since then therapies, equipment, monitoring devices and management have improved in hundreds of ways. Real-time home blood glucose monitoring is routine, human insulin has been synthesized and pump technology perfected. The work continues to offer diabetics ever-improving lifestyles and life expectancies that were impossible as recently as the 1920's.

Even with great care diabetes is no walk in the park. But thanks to researchers over the centuries, we now truly have a fighting chance to live, and live well.

Chapter 2

Similar Symptoms, Different Causes

B oth Type 1 and Type 2 diabetics have high levels of sugar (also called glucose) in the blood. The glucose is a product of digestion, which breaks food down into sugar that is put into the bloodstream for distribution throughout the body. Despite an overabundance of sugar in the blood, the body is unable to use it for nourishment so it builds up in the bloodstream.

This inability causes two things to happen:

- The body's cells can't use the glucose so they starve.
- Excessive sugar in the blood causes damage to your body.

The potential complications are the same in both types. Sustained high blood glucose levels (BGLs) can weaken and clog blood vessels over time while also damaging the kidneys, eyes, feet, heart, blood vessels, nerves, skin and bones. It may also increase the chances of Alzheimer's disease, stroke, osteoporosis and hearing impairment.

Let's look at what happens. When a normal person eats, the food is digested into glucose and the bloodstream carries it to the body's cells. When it gets there a hormone called insulin "unlocks" the cells and allows the glucose to enter so the cells can absorb it for nourishment. The pancreas produces the right amount of insulin for the glucose in the blood in a finely tuned dance. By doing this the body automatically keeps the blood glucose level (BGL) in a narrow healthy range.

It's an amazing system. Candy and junk food obviously contain lots of sugar. But healthy foods raise the BGL too—potato does it big time, even before you load on the fixin's. Carbohydrates, which the body converts into glucose, are all over the place—bread, beans, fruit, pasta, corn, salad dressings and tons of other places you may not think of. Whatever a non-diabetic person eats, their body automatically produces the right amount of insulin for it, their cells allow the insulin to work so they absorb the glucose from the blood, and the BGL is kept in balance.

In both types of diabetes this process is short-circuited and glucose is left circulating in the bloodstream, causing a high BGL. The body reacts by generating thirst, driving you to put fluids into your body that will be expelled and carry excess sugar from the bloodstream with it. That's why the term diabetes mellitus ("honeysweet urination") mentioned in Chapter 1 applies to both types. They both result in high BGLs and the resultant expelling of sugar in the urine. But this is essentially where the similarity between Type 1 and Type 2 ends.

Type 1 diabetes is an autoimmune disease in which the body's own defenses turn against the insulin-producing cells in the pancreas. The cells are killed, wrecking the pancreas's ability to produce insulin. When a Type 1 eats, glucose enters the bloodstream but the insulin doesn't get produced to enable the body to use it. The unused glucose stays in the blood.

In Type 2 the pancreas initially works fine. It senses rising BGLs and produces insulin just like a non-diabetic person. The problem here is called "insulin resistance" because many of the body's cells don't allow insulin to unlock them. When a Type 2 eats, the glucose enters the bloodstream and the pancreas produces insulin. But the insulin resistant cells have barred the doors and the sugar stays in the bloodstream.

Insulin resistance doesn't trigger the Type 2 diagnosis all by itself. Because the body's cells get increasingly more insulin resistant, the pancreas works ever harder to produce enough insulin to overcome it. Eventually many of the overworked insulin producing cells die, the ability of the pancreas to produce insulin is compromised and high BGLs result. So the immediate cause of a diabetes diagnosis is insufficient insulin production but the underlying cause is insulin resistance that may have been present for years.

The high BGLs caused by both types can wreak havoc with your body over the long term. But the good news is that with modern equipment and therapies, diabetics have the tools to effectively control their BGLs and prevent or forestall complications. And even if complications occur, modern treatments can prevent blindness, amputation and other extreme consequences if caught early on.

A number of potential complications are caused by chronically high blood sugar. The feet are one example. Since they're the furthest parts of the body from the heart, if circulation problems develop they're likely to show up there first. The feet can get nerve damage, called neuropathy, that can cause pain, tingling or a numbness that impairs the ability to feel heat, cold and pain. This increases the possibility of having an injury that could go unnoticed. At the same time, the healing process may be weakened and that increases the chance of infection. An infection is bad enough for non-diabetics; in diabetics it's a major league threat that can lead to amputation if it gets out of hand.

Because of this, foot problems must be addressed quickly. If you ask a podiatrist for a diabetic horror story, they'll usually tell you about the person who came in with a gangrenous foot that required amputation. They furrow their brows, get really serious and quietly say, "Why didn't they see me earlier?" Since foot problems like infections can be immediately threatening, podiatrists will see you on the day you call if they know you're diabetic.

In the old days blindness was a frequent untreatable complication of diabetes. The most common eye disease among diabetics is called diabetic retinopathy. A number of bad things can happen as a result of the condition. One is the leakage of blood from weak blood vessels that can cloud the center of the eye and block vision.

Eye problems are sneaky because there aren't obvious symptoms before trouble starts. That's why it's important to have to have a comprehensive dilated eye exam at least annually. It can identify potential problems early so they can be addressed before the vision is impaired.

Diabetics need to be aware of their bodies and avoid letting conditions get out hand. It's part of the routine, just like BGL management. Today's medical technology can treat many of the serious consequences that used to be inevitable, and doctors are blown away when patients show up too late for them to help.

Regardless of which type you have, higher than normal BGLs will happen for most of us no matter how tightly we try to control it. This makes it even more important to control cholesterol and blood pressure, and your doctor may prescribe medications for either or both. The standards for each are tighter for diabetic patients because of the higher levels of glucose already floating in our bloodstreams. Both high cholesterol levels and blood pressure are dangerous for everyone; if you add in high blood sugar the potential for trouble increases dramatically. And smoking adds another level of risk that compounds the chances of complications even more.

Carbohydrates have a big impact since they're broken down into glucose that enters the bloodstream. Diabetics can eat anything but need to be aware of how much. For example, macaroni and cheese—a high carb dish—may be fine for your growing kids but you'll find if you eat much of it your BGL will spike. Small amounts are OK, but other foods with less carbohydrate are better choices. There are a number of ways to control diet and nutritionists can help develop individual strategies.

Perhaps the most important thing both types have in common is the effect of exercise. My medical professional once told me that of all the diabetics in her practice, regardless of which type, the ones who are successful in controlling it all exercise regularly—and not just in spurts. Think about it— you've got glucose in your bloodstream that wants to build up on the vessel walls. Is it more likely to do it in a slow-moving, sedentary bloodstream or in a fast-moving, active one? It's not rocket science.

The symptoms, complications, some of the management practices and the need for BGL balance are common to both Type 1 and Type 2. But they're fundamentally different diseases with markedly different treatment strategies, as we'll see.

Chapter 3
Type 1

Type 1 diabetes occurs when the pancreas makes little or no insulin. Although it usually strikes young people, it can happen at any time of life. I got it when I was 29.

If you've gotten this diagnosis it's not the end of the world, but you'll find life has changed in ways that can be confusing and even overwhelming. Sometimes it can also be depressing as you realize the practical impact it has on your everyday life. Once you understand the way the elements of control (mainly diet/insulin/exercise) work together, you'll have the ability to control your BGLs. Diabetes affects people differently and you need to customize your treatment to your (and I mean *your*) body. You'll be able to live a full and long life, but how long and how full will partly depend on how successfully you manage the disease.

What Happened?

Your immune system normally defends your body against harmful bacteria, viruses and other things. When it senses the presence of the invaders, it produces specialized antibodies to destroy the threat. For unknown reasons your immune system turned on your body, attacked the insulin producing cells in your pancreas and killed them. This crippled your ability to produce insulin.

Insulin's job is to unlock the body's cells so sugar can get in to provide nourishment. Without it, glucose couldn't enter the cells and it built up in your bloodstream.

The kidneys tried to get rid of the excess glucose, which is why you urinated so often. Your body needed to replace the fluids it was expelling, so you were compelled to drink by that unstoppable thirst. In the meantime, because your body couldn't use the glucose in your blood you were slowly starving. That's why you lost weight regardless of how much you ate. The high BGL also made you feel listless and tired.

Why Me?

There are a number of risk factors for Type 1, but the actual cause isn't known. Having parents or siblings with diabetes indicates a higher risk (my youngest brother has had Type 1 longer than me). Ethnicity can be a risk factor—there are higher rates in people of Northern European descent, with Scandinavians having the highest incidence.

You may have increased risk if your mother was younger than 25 when she had you, had preeclampsia while pregnant or if you were born jaundiced. The same goes for those who had a respiratory infection shortly after birth. Another risk factor is having a low level of Vitamin D, but drinking cow's milk—the common source of Vitamin D—early in life apparently raises the risk.

We know that some environmental factor triggers the auto-immune problem, and it's possible viruses are the cause. Although a link hasn't been conclusively proven, many Type 1's remember getting really sick sometime before they were diagnosed. In any case, the pancreas's production of insulin is crippled. Interestingly, the pancreas continues to grow more islet cells, but the immune system gets increasingly good at killing them off. The result is the same—insufficient insulin production.

There are lots of clues but no real answers. Two things are for sure—there's no magic bullet to prevent the disease and you can't blame yourself for getting it.

The Importance of Balance

Non-diabetics automatically maintain their blood glucose in the normal range. Whatever they eat and however much they exercise (or don't) their pancreases know how much insulin is needed and crank out just the right amount. The body's cells absorb the glucose, the insulin is used up and the BGL stays in the normal range.

Since Type 1's don't produce their own insulin they must inject it (digestion breaks insulin down, so taking it orally doesn't work). The question is, "how much and when," and the answer is not only complicated but it can change over the course of a day.

Diabetics need to think like a pancreas and administer the correct amount of insulin for the amount of food eaten and the effect of exercise or other factors. If we misjudge we wind up with BGLs that are too high or low and there are consequences for each.

The Short Term Danger of High BGLs

When a body can't get nourishment because of a lack of insulin, it gets creative. It turns on itself and breaks down its own fats to get energy. Here's the problem—the process produces acids called ketones that can build up in the bloodstream and poison the body.

There are signs when this happens, ranging from the familiar symptoms of a high BGL to difficulty in breathing, a fruity odor on the breath, confusion and nausea. Fortunately, it develops slowly and a person experiencing it has time to get to a hospital for help. But it must be treated.

Mega-bestselling author Anne Rice ignored her symptoms, which included weight loss, an inability to concentrate or write, and strange behavior. She finally collapsed into a coma. A nurse couldn't find a pulse and she was rushed to a hospital where her BGL was over 800 (normal is 70-130). She came within a whisker of dying.

It's called diabetic ketoacidosis (DKA) and it's deadly serious—left untreated it is fatal. It's the endgame of untreated diabetes that was the inevitable fate of Type 1 diabetics before insulin became available.

The Long Term Effects of High BGLs

In the long run, chronically high BGLs can result in really bad stuff like kidney disease, blindness, heart disease that can lead to heart attacks or strokes, and amputations. Other complications include impaired balance and nerve damage that can cause numbness, a "pins and needles" sensation and shooting pains. There are more, but you get the point.

That's the bad news. The good news is that with today's medical technology we've got the tools to avoid them and when they do occur we can treat many of them. For example, laser eye surgery is a painless procedure done in the office that can prevent blindness.

The Immediate Threat of Low BGLs

There are different terms for low blood sugar reactions. These include reaction, shock, hypoglycemic shock, insulin reaction, low sugar reaction, hypoglycemic reaction, and diabetic shock. They all mean the same thing.

Reactions are serious business, because when the BGL goes too low it affects the brain cells. Unlike other cells in the body, brain cells don't store glucose so when there isn't enough in the bloodstream to fuel them they go haywire. Since the brain controls the body's functions all kinds of things start to go wrong.

The symptoms vary from person to person, but can include loss of mental acuity, poor coordination, dizziness, shakiness, blurry vision, rapid heartbeat, sweating, fatigue, nervousness and unconsciousness. Others can include irrational behavior and utter helplessness. It's dangerous because if symptoms like foggy thinking, dizziness, poor coordination and unconsciousness occur at a bad time—like when you're driving—the consequences can be ugly.

Just ask Ricky Jones, who had a reaction and crashed his car. When the responding police officer ordered him to get out of the vehicle, Jones was unresponsive. The officer saw this as a refusal to cooperate and shot him with a Taser twice before EMT's diagnosed his low BGL.

As serious as reactions can be, they're easy to treat before they get out of hand. The most important thing is to know what your symptoms are, because they vary from person to person and change over time. I may be the only person in history whose low BGL causes weakness in the knees—they feel like they're about to buckle when I use the stairs. And if I don't eat sugar promptly they *will* give out. When I feel this way, I don't even check my BGL because I know it's low. Whatever your particular symptoms are, you need to recognize them.

Since the problem is treated with glucose it's important keep sugar handy so you can treat a low BGL before it goes too far. Glucose tablets are great—they're fast acting and come in small containers that fit in your pocket. You should be able to treat low BGLs so quickly and smoothly that others won't even notice. Extreme events like car accidents happen, but they're really rare.

If the worst happens and you can't treat yourself, someone else can give you an emergency injection of glucagon, which stimulates the liver to release glucose. It's a safe way to help because it eliminates the danger of choking that could happen if someone tried to feed you. Here's the trick—whoever responds needs to know where it is and how to use it. If the people with you don't want to administer it, a call to 911 will bring EMT's who'll figure out what's going on quickly. They're familiar with the drill because they see insulin reactions regularly in calls they make all over town.

A Ride in the Ambulance

Reactions can happen for a number of reasons. Taking too much insulin for the food you've eaten or skipping a meal can cause it. Anything that leaves insulin in the blood without enough glucose to act on can reduce the BGL to dangerous levels.

Years ago, after a high-carb day of holiday celebrating I misjudged my food intake and gave myself too much insulin. Way too much. I woke up in the middle of the night to find the bedroom lit up like daytime and several EMT's surrounding the bed. I was incoherent and unable to move. Even though I was the center of attention I was really just an observer with an extremely intimate view of the action. They put me in an ambulance and I laid there on the stretcher watching an EMT fill a giant syringe—it had to be an inch in diameter and 8 inches long. I thought, "man, the needle on the end of that thing must be HUGE." To my relief it just went into an IV line that fed glucose into my bloodstream.

Within minutes I felt better. Exhausted, to be sure, but at least I had my brain back. The amazing thing about insulin reactions is that once you treat them by raising the BGL you recover your mental ability immediately. Here's the hard part. Except for what I've shared here, I still don't remember anything about that night. My wife and sons tell me it was really scary for them because Dad "disappeared." My distressed body was there, but I wasn't. To this day I haven't asked for details and they haven't offered them. That night something else took over and it's important we insulin dependent diabetics work to avoid it.

Severe reactions happen, but they shouldn't occur often. Researchers say they'll happen about two times a year, but I haven't had them nearly that often. Like so much about diabetes, it varies with the individual.

The Nuts and Bolts of Control

Knowing the consequences of high and low BGLs is motivation for keeping good balance, but it can still be hard to do. Great control takes education, effort, commitment and an understanding of the way your own body operates. It can be daunting, but when you develop some knowledge you'll learn to use tools that we could only dream of a few years ago. Insulin is readily available, real-time blood sugars can be determined quickly at home, and the process is probably less painful than you imagine. Good management is more attainable than ever before.

If you want absolutely great control, the best scenario is one where you have the same schedule every day. It would mean standardizing breakfast, exercise, office work, cleaning, lunch, computer work, yard work, socializing, dinner, club meetings, watching TV and an evening snack. If you did the same things in the same measure at the same time every day, you could have really stellar control.

Do you live like this? Do you know anyone who does? The variability of our days is what makes great control as much an art as a science. Your medical professionals can give you all kinds of help, advice and tools, and you absolutely need them. But ultimately it's your job to be aware of your BGLs, adjust for the particular circumstances you have at the time, and manage your own diabetes 24/7/365.

In the years since I was diagnosed there's been a revolutionary change from guessing about our treatment to knowing what we need. Before electronic blood glucose monitoring we checked urine for the presence of sugar by putting a sample on a glucose-sensitive paper strip, but the results were old news. They only showed whether you had been in control earlier when waste (including excess sugar) had been expelled from your body. The yellow tape would turn green if glucose was present and the shade (from light to really dark) would indicate whether you had spilled just a little or a whole lot of glucose. It boiled down to giving yourself an "attaboy" if it stayed yellow or playing a guessing game about how much insulin to take if it was green. We were flying by the seats of our pants and using old information to deduce our actual BGLs.

For years after I was diagnosed I knew when my BGL was going too low because my body readily sensed changes.

One sign I was trending too low was if I started feeling really good. This meant I was passing from a higher BGL down through the normal range (which felt great) on the way further down to a low BGL. I often wondered how great it must be to feel like that all the time—without thinking about when and by how much I'd soon be drifting out of it.

With the blood glucose meters we use today, the realtime BGL can be known immediately, and this has transformed the prospects for tighter control. There's a test called the hemoglobin A1c that shows what your average BGL has been over the previous two to three months. In the days before home metering, an A1c of 8-9 was considered good control. Today the target is under 7.0 and many diabetics achieve it.

Eventually BGL testing and correction becomes routine. It takes less time than brushing your teeth and can be practically painless. Here's how it's done:

1. Put a disposable test strip into the meter.
2. Prick your finger with a lancet to produce a small drop of blood.
3. Apply the blood to the test strip.
4. In a few seconds read your BGL on the meter's digital display.

Knowing your BGL gives you the critical information you need to maintain good control. Another key piece of information is the carbohydrate content of your food. Since carbohydrates are the food components that get digested into sugars it's important to know how much you're consuming. Fortunately they're listed on food packaging and can be found in pocket-sized books that show them for hundreds of items including items served at many restaurants.

BGL and carb content information enable you to take correct immediate action and help you plan ahead for the day. If the BGL is low you can eat carbs to raise it. If it's high you can figure out how much insulin you need to lower it. Before you eat you can calculate how many carbs you'll consume and adjust your insulin ahead of time to keep your BGL in the target range. If you're going to work out you should have an idea of how many carbs you'll burn and eat the right amount of carbohydrate to keep your BGL from bottoming out. It sounds like a lot of figuring, but once you've learned how your body works it becomes second nature.

The blood glucose meter revolutionized diabetic therapy and the development of the insulin pump took it even further. The pump contains a reservoir of insulin it delivers through a tiny plastic tube (called a cannula) placed in your soft tissue. If you do it right—which isn't hard—the insertion is painless. The introducer needle is a hellacious looking thing, so this is hard to believe but true! The cannula is so short, soft and flexible you don't even feel it's there and, best of all, it only needs to be replaced every three days. When you're on the pump, which is a gizmo about the size of a cell phone, individual injections are no longer needed.

With the pump you can give yourself insulin discreetly anytime, anywhere. Out of courtesy for others, when we're using syringes most of us like to find a restroom or other private place to take injections. In practicality this means you sometimes don't take the shot, especially if you only need a small amount. Since the pump lets you administer it unobtrusively simply by pressing buttons there's no need to forgo a dose just because it's inconvenient. The ease of use translates into better control.

Amazingly, when you check your BGL the home glucose meter radios the information to the pump, which puts the data into its computer. It remembers the amount of unused insulin in your body and is able to calculate how much insulin you need to adjust your current BGL. Or, if you enter the amount of carbs you plan to eat, it will tell you how much insulin you need to cover them. It eliminates having to figure out how much insulin you need and provides accuracy that was impossible only a few years ago.

And get this—long–lasting batteries power both the meter and the pump so you can always have the entire system with you to use anytime, anywhere.

Get a Grip

People can get depressed over being diabetic, especially if they're new to it and are coming to realize how much their lives have just changed. I get that, but we should really be thankful to be alive. Type 1 complicates everything, but we can still do just about anything non-diabetics can. Travel and sports are certainly doable. People with diabetes climb tall mountains, play in the National Basketball Association and scuba dive. You can find them at the tops of many professions, but you wouldn't know they have it unless they told you.

United States Supreme Court Justice Sonia Sotomayor has Type 1. So does Chicago Bears quarterback Jay Cutler. Academy Award-winning actress Halle Berry was diagnosed at age 23. Bret Michaels is the lead singer for Poison who won Donald Trump's Celebrity Apprentice, and swimmer Gary Hall won Olympic gold. Millions of people with diabetes quietly manage their condition and pursue excellence as vigorously as anyone else. So can you.

Chapter 4

Type 1 Kids

Laura Maloney-Hastillo was on a business trip when she received the 1:00 AM call. Her 2-1/2 year old son Caleb had been brought to the ER. He hadn't been feeling well, which was unusual for him, and he was drinking a lot. Since everybody figured he had a stomach bug his frequent consumption of ginger ale seemed to be a good thing. But he didn't improve and now he was in the hospital where a blood test showed his BGL was over 800, putting him in diabetic ketoacidosis (DKA). Caleb was severely dehydrated and the staff had trouble finding a blood vessel to put an IV into. When it was finally installed they were able to give him fluids for rehydration. That was good news—until the doctor told Laura, "I need you to hear me—we're not out of the woods yet." There was still a good chance he would fall into a coma. Two hours later she clambered onto the next flight out of Kansas City to Connecticut for an excruciating trip home. Things turned out OK—after two days in the PICU and three more in the hospital, Caleb was in shape to go home.

Laura had suspicions about diabetes for about two months before the diagnosis and had spoken to the pediatrician's office about it more than once. Caleb was drinking obsessively—he was even drinking bath water. She was told that the constant drinking wasn't unusual for two-year-olds and as long as there wasn't any diabetes in the family she had nothing to worry about.

The diagnosis was made 1½ years ago. Caleb is cute as a button with blonde hair, hazel eyes and an infectious smile. He remembers his ordeal like it was a fun outing—he got to sleep in a cage (the hospital crib) and ate goldfish crackers! He's a very smart kid who loves Michael Jackson, dancing, candy and "Rufus," the bear with diabetes he got from the Juvenile Diabetes Research Foundation.

The JDRF's mission is to cure the disease but it's also a repository of practical information for diabetics of any age, including kids who have Type 1 and their parents. Among many other things, it hosts a web page called Real Talk where kids can share their stories with each other. For example, it's a forum for 12 year-old Jade Gamber who wrote a book called *I've Got a Secret* about her experiences—good and bad—with Type 1. At first she was reluctant to tell her story but came to feel it could help others. She says "Some of it is personal and a little embarrassing, but I know it will help other kids who have diabetes and feel scared."

Life changed for everyone in Caleb's family. Laura understood the seriousness of the condition but also recognized how little she knew about it, so she immersed herself in diabetes education. Laura has to deal with Caleb's blood sugar balance just as adult diabetics do, but she's one step removed. Unable to experience the symptoms herself, she needs to keep an eagle eye on her son to try to figure out what's going on with his BGLs. Even adult diabetics who live with their own symptoms can have trouble with control. Just imagine the difficulty of managing it for someone else as an observer.

These are some of the things she has to deal with:

- Giving Caleb insulin to cover the meal he's eating and then having him shrug off the food after three bites.
- Checking his BGL to find it inexplicably high, only to find out he sneaked a snack earlier.
- Watching for mood and physical changes that might indicate a low BGL and checking his BGL quickly if low sugar is suspected.

Laura is committed to excellence in caring for her son. To get advice, she once attended a support group for parents of diabetic kids but sensed that some group members were overreacting by waking their kids up several times a night to check their BGLs. She found that by letting her son go to bed with a slightly higher BGL they could both get a good night's sleep.

Parents want the best for their children, but sometimes the cure is worse than the disease. Everybody needs sleep and not getting enough can lead to health problems, even in dedicated moms. And the kids, who spend more time in deep-sleep than adults, shouldn't be deprived of it either. In the end, Laura figured out that constant night-time monitoring was counterproductive for all concerned and she found ways to adjust that helped everyone lead a closer to normal life.

But it's not normal. All parents need to watch their young ones, but not with the same intensity. The balance between food, exercise and insulin can be hard to control for a couple of reasons. First, the effect of a child's high energy activity is harder to peg. Second, typical childhood fussiness about what they eat and how much can throw carb-counting out the window. Together they make insulin calculations harder than it is for adults.

It affects life in unexpected ways. Caleb doesn't like to go to bed, so he'll say he needs a blood test, because he knows his mom won't put him in bed if she thinks his BGL might be low. Sibling rivalries being what they are, giving Caleb candy to treat a low BGL is an opportunity for one-upmanship over his brother, Levi, who isn't allowed to eat as much candy. Sending him to a friend's house without someone knowledgeable about diabetes is out of the question.

Finding a babysitter was hard until Laura asked the school nurse if she knew of a responsible diabetic high school student who would like to do it. It was a great idea—she found Daniel, who the whole family has come to adore. The first time he watched the boys Laura realized how completely he understood Type 1. And was so relieved she cried.

The demands of supervising Type 1 kids are serious. They made sending Caleb to Pre-K terrifying and preclude sending him on play dates at other kid's houses. Despite the pain and inconvenience Type 1 brings, she tries to watch what she says because she never wants her son to feel like a burden.

No matter how hard a caregiver tries, there will be times when the BGL gets out of control and you'll never figure out why. Sometimes you may think you've got a handle on it—just before a two-inch growth spurt changes everything. You've been given an incredibly difficult task and you can only do your best.

You've got tools that are double-edged swords. On one hand, you can know your child's BGL in minutes and take appropriate action immediately. On the other hand the information triggers an underlying emotional guilt trip: "He's too high! He's too low! How could I let this happen?" You beat yourself up over something you'll never be able to perfectly control.

My friend Deb Ciosek was diagnosed at age 6 and lived on one injection a day for twenty years. Today she has exquisite control using current technology and can't imagine how she made it through the early years without it. But at least Deb's mom was free from the constant stress of high tech monitoring and control. Her underlying emotion was simpler: "Thank God for insulin. My daughter has hope!"

Most diabetics aren't Deb, who is one of around 1500 people alive today who have had diabetes for over 50 years. There may be something about her metabolism that enabled her to survive better than most. Please don't think that Deb's longevity, which was achieved despite the rudimentary control she had for those many years, is an excuse to forgo the tight control that's possible today. You may not have whatever unknown thing she has going for her.

The point is that this is a difficult situation and parents/caregivers shouldn't punish themselves unnecessarily if they don't achieve the clinical ideal. Dealing with diabetes is a relentless marathon full of ups, downs and unexpected twists and there will be times when you simply can't figure out why something happened.

Actually, a marathon is a wholly inadequate metaphor. It's demanding and relentless, for sure. But after 26.2 miles there's a finish line.

There's got to be a special place in heaven for responsible parents and caregivers of diabetic children.

Chapter 5

Prediabetes

Prediabetes is a warning shot telling you that Type 2 diabetes may be in your future, especially if you don't take steps to avoid it. People figure prediabetics have some vague factors at work that may or may not cause them to develop diabetes, and they often think it just means you should lose some weight. If only it was that simple.

The underlying cause of prediabetes is insulin resistance, the same as in full-blown Type 2. The difference between them is the blood sugar level (BGL). A fasting normal BGL is under 100 mg/dl and the threshold for a Type 2 diagnosis is 126 or higher. Prediabetes occupies the middle ground between 100 and 126: too high to be normal but too low to be Type 2.

Prediabetics can avoid a diagnosis of Type 2 by keeping their BGLs under 126. This can often be accomplished with diet, exercise and weight control. Here's why:

Insulin acts as a key to unlock your body's cells so they'll accept glucose from the bloodstream for nourishment. When the cells become insulin resistant, your body needs more insulin to unlock them. Initially, your pancreas rises to the occasion and produces the extra insulin. But over time the overworked insulin producing cells (called beta cells) gradually die and the pancreas can't keep up with the demand. At this point the BGL can rise to diabetic levels.

The challenge for prediabetics is to minimize the burden on the pancreas and conserve its ability to work effectively. This is where diet, exercise and weight control come into play.

Watching your diet can reduce the amount of glucose you put into your bloodstream in the first place, which reduces the need for insulin. Exercise has two major benefits. First, it decreases overall insulin resistance so less insulin is required to unlock the cells. Second, physical activity enables muscle cells to absorb glucose from the bloodstream without needing insulin to do so. Because of this, an elevated BGL can be knocked down by exercise without overtaxing the beta cells. Losing weight reduces the number of cells needing insulin and this consequently reduces the demands on your pancreas.

By using diet/exercise/weight control, prediabetics can forestall and even prevent the higher BGLs that indicate Type 2. This regimen also improves blood pressure, cholesterol and the effectiveness of diabetic medications that may be prescribed. Diet/exercise/weight control is the cornerstone of prediabetic treatment for good reason.

Insulin resistance is progressive and around 70% of those with prediabetes will develop Type 2. Those who forgo an effective program to control it are certainly in this group. But 30% of prediabetics won't be. There is no cure for insulin resistance, but with proper care, discipline and persistence, it can be managed so that Type 2 is delayed or avoided.

Chapter 6
Type 2

There are several other kinds of diabetes that can arise for a variety of medical reasons. But the Type 2 version is responsible for 90-95% of all cases so we'll focus on it. It used to be called "Adult Onset Diabetes" because it typically struck later in life, but Type 2 has now become epidemic even among young people.

Some think Type 2 is less serious than Type 1, but this is untrue. High blood sugar is damaging regardless of which type caused it and both types can be hard to control.

What Happened?

Your body's cells stopped behaving normally and became resistant to a hormone called insulin. When you eat, food is broken down into glucose that enters your bloodstream and is carried to cells for nourishment. Insulin's job is to "unlock" the cells and allow glucose to enter, but your cells developed insulin resistance. When insulin was unable to unlock the cells, glucose couldn't enter and it remained in the bloodstream.

Unlike in Type 1, where most or all of the insulin-producing cells (called beta cells) have been destroyed, your pancreas continued to produce insulin. It actually worked harder to produce even more insulin than normal in attempting to overcome the insulin resistance. By the time you were diagnosed with Type 2, your beta cells were stressed and over half had died. Insulin production decreased, insulin resistance increased and high BGLs resulted.

Type 2 develops gradually and often sneaks up on people. It can take up to ten years for diabetes to develop, and the incremental changes along the way are easy to miss. It's like the old story about boiling a frog—if you suddenly drop him into hot water he'll sense the change and jump out, but if you raise the temperature a little at a time he won't know he's in trouble until it's too late.

Type 2 can be like this. Because they're unaware of the small incremental changes, people don't realize they've got diabetes. It's estimated that at least 25% of diabetics don't even know they have it. Many people only discover it through a routine screening, often after damage has been done.

Why Me?

Scientists don't know why Type 2 strikes some people and not others, but there are some factors that indicate increased risk. Some are beyond our control, but others aren't. Here are some:

- A family history of diabetes
- Being over 40 years old
- Having Latino, African American, Native American, Asian American or Pacific Island heritage
- A diagnosis of prediabetes
- High blood pressure
- Abnormal cholesterol levels

Excessive weight and sedentary lifestyles can cause inflammation that worsens insulin resistance, but we don't know why insulin resistance happens in the first place. It's not limited to inactive overweight people—active thin people also get it and many obese people don't.

But excess weight does increase the odds and researchers believe there's something causative at work in overweight people even though it's not yet understood.

The Nuts and Bolts of Control

There are a number of ways to control Type 2. The first steps are diet, exercise and weight control, which you may have already used to treat prediabetes. Even after diabetes is diagnosed, the same benefits of diet, exercise and weight control apply. Moderate exercise enables your cells to use glucose at as much as 20 times the normal rate by revving up your metabolism and reducing insulin resistance, and diet can help control the amount of glucose you put into your bloodstream in the first place.

Dropping weight by just 5—7% can reduce insulin resistance, blood pressure, cholesterol, and the BGL. All of them are keys to your long term health. The amazing thing is you don't need to train for a triathlon or fit into your high school jeans—just walking and diet changes can pay off big time. Type 2 diabetes is a progressive disease and this strategy can help stop it or slow it down. Here's the hard truth—if you don't exercise and control your weight, the severity can develop faster and complications can come sooner.

As long as diet and exercise work, they are the best therapy. But in most cases of Type 2, insulin resistance increases and insulin production decreases to the point where diet, exercise and weight control aren't enough and medication is needed.

Oral medicines are often prescribed to help control Type 2. The four basic classes of medications each do different things.

They can:

1. Help the body's cells use insulin more effectively by decreasing insulin resistance.
2. Stimulate the pancreas to increase insulin production.
3. Decrease the amount of sugar released by the liver.
4. Block stomach enzymes to reduce the sugar released through digestion.

Injectable non-insulin medications can also help lower blood glucose. The two classes can do either of the following:

1. Slow down food absorption, help you feel full and reduce glucose production by the liver.
2. Help suppress your appetite and lower the BGL after meals.

Medications from different classes can be used simultaneously, and some are used together so regularly they're combined into one tablet. For example, Glucovance tablets contain metformin (to reduce sugar production in the liver and make cellular insulin receptors more sensitive) and glyburide (to stimulate release of insulin by the pancreas). There are a variety of brand name drugs within each class that come in different strengths and they can be used in a huge number of combinations. Since diabetes varies so much between people, medication requirements can vary dramatically from person to person.

Diabetes is unlike other conditions where patients can take "one size fits all" medication and then passively let it work. Prescribing the correct combinations and dosages for Type 2 is much more complex. This is partly because the effectiveness of the medications is dependent on things beyond your doctor's control, like your lifestyle. And this is where your active effort is necessary.

Look at it this way—if your doctor could count on you to maintain your weight, consume the same diet on the same schedule every day, never get sick, maintain a rigid daily exercise routine where you burn the same amount of carbohydrates each time, and do all of it while remaining stress-free, he'd have a better shot at precisely prescribing the right medications.

We all know this isn't going to happen, but the point is that the more you standardize diet and exercise the better chance you have of controlling your BGL. If you routinely swing from a high carb to a low carb diet or have an erratic exercise routine, you're burying your doctor with variables he can't account for. He can't effectively prescribe medication when your behavior makes you a moving target. Finding the right treatment mix (diet, exercise and medication) involves trial and error based on your individual characteristics, so close communication with your medical professional is critical.

The less you stabilize diet and exercise, the harder it is to determine effective medications. Here are three scenarios that assume the same medications in the same strengths are taken at the proper times. In the first, you stick to your diet and exercise schedule. You feel great because your BGL is in a good range. In the second, you overeat and then nod off. Glucose rises in your bloodstream because of the excess food and it stays high because you haven't burned it off through activity. You feel sluggish and out of sorts due to your high BGL. Third, you work or play physically and haven't taken time to eat. Your BGL drops too much and, depending on your medication, you may experience a low blood sugar reaction.

In real life your daily behavior can be any of these or a combination somewhere in between. The point is this—think about what you're doing and work to limit large swings in your BGL. The effort will pay off—you'll feel better and your long term health will improve.

Your doctor will probably recommend checking your BGL regularly. If it's high some immediate steps can be taken, like being careful about what else you eat and getting some exercise. Not only will activity reduce insulin resistance but your muscles will use glucose in the blood for energy. Both factors can help lower your BGL.

If your tests indicate chronically high BGLs, you should see your medical professional to change things and get it back under control. Remember, it's a progressive disease that will probably change over time and periodic adjustments will need to be made.

If you can't control your BGL with the medications described earlier, insulin injections may be necessary. While there's often a knee-jerk aversion to the idea, it may be the only way to control your BGL. If your doctor prescribes insulin the chances are your pancreas may have reached a point that where it can't be coaxed to produce enough insulin and, as a result, your BGLs are chronically high and will stay that way without more help.

I've got Type 1 and when people find out I take insulin they sometimes lower their voices, get a sympathetic look in their eyes, and say, "So, you've got it really bad." The fact is that both types are serious whether you use insulin or not and if you've got them at all you've got something "bad."

You or your loved ones may feel the same way when insulin is prescribed. It's true that your diabetes has reached a new plateau and some changes are needed to manage it. But insulin is just a new (to you) effective tool to help keep your BGL in balance. Up to this point you've already been fighting to stay on the tightrope and that's the hard part. That battle won't go away but the chances are it will be easier with insulin therapy.

Insulin is very safe, it will definitely reduce your BGLs, you'll be able to take as much as you need and it won't become ineffective over time. It's common to resist taking insulin; it's also common for diabetics who try it to immediately feel better and wonder why they ever fought it.

If a Type 2 uses insulin, it doesn't mean he's become a Type 1. He's still got insulin resistance, which is the hallmark of Type 2 but isn't present in Type 1. He'll just be using a different therapy that also happens to be used in Type 1.

Insulin therapy works, but it brings issues that many Type 2's haven't had to deal with. If you'd like to know more about using insulin please read the chapter on Type 1.

Can Type 2's Experience Low Blood Sugar Reactions?

Yes, but many don't know it and are mystified when they experience them. The symptoms of a low BGL can be sweating, a cold clammy feeling, dizziness, shakiness, weakness, irritability, hunger, nervousness, paleness, rapid heartbeat, blurry vision, confusion or others. They vary from person to person and people can have one or a combination of them.

Low blood sugar (hypoglycemia) can be dangerous if it goes too low at a bad time. For example, you wouldn't want to be dizzy and shaky with blurry vision while climbing a ladder, so it's important diabetics learn to recognize it and treat it. Fortunately, it's easily corrected by taking a glucose tablet, drinking orange juice or ingesting sugar in other ways.

Some Type 2 medications can promote hypoglycemia by themselves and others will do it in combination with other diabetic or non-diabetic treatments. Some seemingly innocuous drugs—like aspirin—can lower the BGL. Alcohol can too.

Unexpectedly delaying eating—like when a restaurant keeps you waiting longer than you planned—may allow your medications to bring the BGL down too much. The same is true if you exercise longer or more strenuously than expected. A Type 2 told me he was once in a softball game for longer than he anticipated and realized he was having a reaction when the playing field became wavy. Diabetics need to have candy or glucose tablets handy for unexpected situations like these.

If you have a chronic problem with low sugar reactions it's important to review your program with your health care professional. You need to keep your BGLs low, but continually flirting with very low BGLs is a bad idea—it can be dangerous if you have a reaction at a time when mental sharpness is important.

The Importance of Balance

Type 2's need to keep their BGLs in balance for the same reasons as Type 1's, but the mechanics are different. Medications change the way your body operates. They can increase functions (by making it easier for cells to use insulin or stimulating the pancreas) or decrease them (by reducing the amounts of glucose released by the liver or the digestive system). Whatever medication or combination of medications you use, they operate together with diet, exercise and other elements—like stress—to determine your BGL. Stress levels may be beyond your control but diet and exercise aren't. If you standardize whatever variables you can, you'll improve your chances for good control.

Real life can interfere with your routine. You might plan to exercise but a "must do now" task crops up. Or, you might be casually enjoying coffee with some friends when those little pastries become irresistible. Or, you may have overslept and in the panic to get out the door you forgot to take your medication.

Life happens, and you're not immune from it just because you're supposed to have a controlled lifestyle. When you're thrown off track and have a high BGL, get it back under control and don't stress out over it. You're striving to keep your average long term BGLs in check and temporary lapses won't keep you from achieving it. Nobody I know of has flawless control and the chances are you won't be perfect either. All any of us can do is the best we can.

Because it varies so much by individual, effective therapy can be as much an art as a science. Paying attention to the way your body responds to diet/medication/exercise and giving feedback to your medical professional is essential in developing the right treatment strategy.

A healthy dose of patience helps, too.

Chapter 7

Vital Signs

The standard vital signs are temperature, pulse, blood pressure and respiratory rate. They're used to check major body functions and are routine parts of medical examinations. BGL data ranks right up with these as a vital sign for diabetics.

I remember my 9th grade biology class when the teacher did a lesson on the blood. I don't recall what we were supposed to learn, but it involved getting your own sample by pricking your finger with a hand-held lancet. The sharp end came to a razor-sharp v-shaped point. It took a few minutes to overcome the "chicken out at the last moment" syndrome but, in an act of stunning bravery, I plunged the sharp into my finger and drew a drop of blood.

Like most diabetic technology, the process has been refined. Happily, today you can put a lancet with a very fine point into a spring-loaded lancing device that restricts the depth. You hold it against your finger and press a trigger button to release it. It's quick and you just feel a slight pinch. This is the only "traumatic" element of BGL testing—which means the whole thing is no big deal as far as pain goes.

This simple process can tell us what our BGL is at that moment. It has eliminated guesswork and given us the ability to control our BGLs by making correct adjustments based on actual data in real time. In addition, if we log our BGLs we can see if we're having large swings between highs and lows.

If we see this is happening we should try to even them out and stabilize the BGL as much as possible.

But individual BGLs only show part of the story because they don't tell us how good our long-term control has been. Even if you kept track of all your BGLs you couldn't accurately calculate this because carbohydrate consumption, exercise and insulin infusion would affect what happened between tests, and the tests probably wouldn't be done at standard time intervals. In the real world determining your average BGL this way isn't practical. This is where the A1c comes in.

The A1c (also called the hemoglobin A1C, HbA1c or glycated hemoglobin) is a blood test that shows your average BGL over the previous two to three months. Hemoglobin is a component of red blood cells that excess sugar in the bloodstream sticks to. The glucose stays with the hemoglobin for the whole life of the cell, and this "glycated hemoglobin" is what the A1c measures. The more glycated hemoglobin you have, the higher your average blood sugar has been.

The A1c is usually done as part of a routine blood test at least each six months, but it may be needed more often. It's an essential tool that shows how successful you've been at managing the whole picture—it's the combined result of medication, diet, exercise and other factors. Your individual metering results are like the tests and quizzes we took in school; the A1c is the final grade.

The following chart shows how an A1c converts to an estimated average BGL.

A1c %	Estim Avg BGL (mg/dl)
5	97
5.5	111
6	126
6.5	140
7	154
7.5	169
8	183
8.5	197
9	212
9.5	226
10	240
10.5	255
11	269
11.5	283
12	298

The American Diabetes Association's general recommendation for the A1c test is less than 7%. This is a good number for diabetics, but even this level results in a higher than normal estimated average BGL, showing an average of 154 mg/dl compared to the normal range of 70-130. Many people don't even come close to 7.0 and it's amazing how high the amount of sugar can be at the higher numbers. The higher the number, the greater the risk of complications.

The A1c isn't just a sterile number. It's a sobering indicator of how much excessive glucose is floating in your blood. And it's a stark reminder that high cholesterol and smoking—both of which add to the debris in your bloodstream—are especially dangerous for diabetics.

Chapter 8

Liver Games

Just when we think we understand what's going on a new complication crops up. We know we need to control our carbohydrate intake because it becomes glucose in the bloodstream. But it turns out food is just one of two main sources of glucose. The other is the liver.

The liver is the biggest organ in the body and it performs around 500 diverse operations. One is to store glucose for later release when the BGL is low. Another is to synthesize glucose from the body's fats and proteins when the liver's reserve of glucose has been exhausted.

The process in non-diabetics is amazing—the pancreas produces insulin to reduce high BGLs and the liver releases glucose to raise low BGLs. It's like having a gyroscope on the tightrope—no matter what you do, you automatically stay balanced. In a normally functioning body this nonstop dance keeps the BGL in a narrow, healthy range.

But diabetes wrecks the ability of the pancreas to keep up its end of the bargain. The liver continues to release glucose when the BGL is low, but if it overshoots the mark the pancreas is unable to produce the insulin to counter it. This raises the BGL.

A question comes to mind. If the liver automatically delivers glucose when the BGL is low, why do we ever have low sugar reactions? One reason is the liver's limited storage capacity. When this is depleted the liver can't respond quickly to a BGL that's dropping due to excess insulin (which can be present in diabetics because it's been injected or caused by some Type 2 medications).

A normal pancreas curtails insulin production when the BGL drops, but diabetes medications don't have kill switches that turn them off when the blood sugar is low. They continue to work regardless of what the BGL is and if the liver doesn't have enough glucose to release, the result is a low BGL we need to fix by eating fast acting carbs.

The liver can throw a monkey wrench into the treatment of both Type 1 and Type 2. Two of its antics, the dawn phenomenon and the Somogyi effect, happen when we're sleeping.

All people experience the "dawn phenomenon," where the liver automatically releases glucose each morning between 4:00 a.m. and 8:00 a.m. to help get the body ready for the day. In non-diabetics the glucose infusion is counteracted by insulin released by the pancreas, which keeps the BGL in the normal range.

But unless a diabetic deliberately supplies the insulin, the liver's action raises the BGL. You'd think we could plan for this, but the amount of glucose released by the liver can vary from day to day even if diet and exercise remain the same. It's hard to anticipate, especially since it's happening before most of us are awake.

The "Somogyi Effect" describes the reaction of the liver to low BGLs at night. It happens if you take too much insulin, don't eat enough food or do anything else that drops your BGL too low. The liver releases glucose into the bloodstream to raise it, but it can overshoot the actual need and leave you with a high BGL in the morning.

The liver doesn't sleep at night and it doesn't take a break in the daytime, either. Roller coaster buffs enjoy the ride partly because of the adrenaline rush. But adrenaline does more than produce exhilaration—it prompts the liver to release glucose to energize the body. The liver senses the adrenaline, figures you're in the "fight or flight" mode and cranks out the sugar it thinks you need to handle the crisis. It immediately raises the BGL even if you haven't eaten anything. It's just another curveball thrown in the liver games.

We can control medication, diet and exercise, but the the liver plays by different rules. The releases of glucose often happen when we're asleep, the amounts are hard to anticipate and they can vary even if we control everything else. It's a wild card that can help explain some of the wacky BGLs we can't make sense of otherwise.

Chapter 9

Pregnancy

The 1989 movie *Steel Magnolias* portrays a character's trials with diabetes in a sympathetic, realistic way.It was a successful Hollywood production that left a big audience with the impression that pregnancy is a bad idea for diabetics.

In the past, before we had the tools that enable tight BGL control, the possibilities for bad outcomes were so serious that doctors often advised against pregnancy. But technology has changed this and diabetic women can now safely become biological moms.

But pregnancy is still risky if BGLs aren't tightly controlled. In a nutshell, here's why. If the mother's blood sugars are high the blood carrying the excessive glucose goes into the baby, raising his/her BGL. These can be especially harmful within the first weeks after conception when the heart, brain, lungs and kidneys are being formed. Because of this, and since women may be pregnant for several weeks before they realize it, it's recommended that BGLs be tightly controlled for 2-3 months before the pregnancy begins.

Later on, after the baby's pancreas has developed, it can make its own insulin and knock down high BGLs received from the mother. But this means the fetus is converting the excess glucose into more energy than it needs, so it's stored as fat. This can result in macrosomia – the medical term for "fat baby." This is serious—the child's shoulders can be damaged during delivery, it may have an excessively low BGL at birth because of their pancreas's overactivity, and the chances of breathing difficulties are greater. They also have a higher risk of obesity and getting Type 2 later on.

Moms can control BGLs better than ever but having diabetes still puts the pregnancy in the high risk category. Lots of women overcome the risk factors and deliver healthy babies. But management is largely up to the mom and if she isn't diligent the impact of high blood sugar is every bit as dangerous today as it ever was.

Doctors check for gestational diabetes in non-diabetic patients later in the pregnancy. As the baby gets larger the mom needs to produce more insulin. If her pancreas isn't able to do this changes must be made to control the BGL. Diet and exercise may be enough, but if they aren't medications may be prescribed. Unlike Types 1 or 2, the gestational variety usually disappears immediately after childbirth, but those who have had it are at greater risk of Type 2 in the future.

Regardless of what kind they have, expectant diabetic women should test their BGLs frequently and take the appropriate action. Type 1's typically struggle with a low BGL during the first trimester due to hormonal changes but find they need to take more insulin in the second and third trimesters. Insulin may be necessary for Type 2's or gestational diabetics.

Any mom – diabetic or not – who conscientiously cares for herself and her baby through pregnancy is a steel magnolia—delicately lovely on the outside but tough as nails underneath.

Diabetes adds a level of difficulty way beyond normal and mothers who handle it successfully are in a different league. They're titanium magnolias.

Chapter 10

Brain Teasers

Both types of diabetes are complicated and our bodies don't always behave the way we think they will. There are lots of situations where unexpected and seemingly illogical things happen. I've had situations I still can't figure out but, luckily, they don't crop up often. Just to give an idea of the kinds of counterintuitive things that can happen, here are a few questions and answers I've stumbled across.

1. **I play competitive softball and don't eat or take insulin beforehand. At the end, after 2 hours of exercise, my BGL is quite a bit higher. Shouldn't it be lower?**

   Studies show that short bursts of activity—like what happens in softball—do temporarily raise blood sugar. But the key word is "temporary;" you need to watch for lows that can happen quite a while after the exercise stops.

2. **My favorite meal is fettucine alfredo with garlic bread, and I feasted on it one night. I counted the carbs, took the insulin, and checked my BGL 2-3 hours later. It was in the desired range. But when I woke up in the morning it was through the roof, even though I didn't eat anything else. Why?**

   Your meal was a combination of carbohydrate and fat. Fat doesn't directly raise the BGL, but it increases free fatty acids

(FFA's) in the bloodstream. FFA's cause insulin resistance, which means it takes more insulin to move sugar from the bloodstream into the cells. Since you only compensated for the carbohydrate content of the meal—and not the FFA's—not enough insulin was taken to overcome the insulin resistance and the glucose remained trapped in the bloodstream. Since fats take longer to digest than carbohydrates, the FFA's kept the BGL high until you took more insulin. That's why the high BGL showed up in the morning.

3. I had a bad cold and was really stuffed up, so I took a decongestant. I rested and ate less than normal to compensate for my lack of activity, but my BGL spiked anyway. What happened?

First of all, just being sick can raise the BGL. On top of this, it's possible the decongestant you took contained pseudoepinephrine or phenylephrine. They open up air passages but can also increase blood sugar. This doesn't happen with everyone, but if you check your BGL after taking the medication and find it has risen, your liver may have reacted to the ingredients (which are related to adrenaline), figured your body was in the fight or flight mode and released glucose for the energy it thought you needed.

Diabetes is full of surprises that don't seem to make sense. Even knowledgeable medical professionals can be thrown off unless careful logs of food consumption, exercise and BGLs are kept. And even then, some situations are hard to figure.

Here's a personal example. I give presentations to groups that last about 45 minutes and I needed to figure out my food/insulin regimen. The idea was to eat enough carbs to keep me from going low while speaking and take enough insulin to keep my BGL from going too high and hurting my mental sharpness. I thought I had it nailed after one presentation that ended with a comfortable BGL of 128.

But the next time the BGL was almost 200 points higher, even though I ate the same amount of carbohydrates and took the same amount of insulin. The only thing that makes sense to me is that the questions and answers in the second session caused a release of adrenaline that raised the BGL. I still follow the same pre-speaking routine, because if I take more insulin to cover the high BGL episode I'll be taking a terrible chance of having a low sugar reaction if the planned-for adrenaline spike doesn't happen. For me, it makes sense to have a temporary high BGL rather than risk bottoming out with a reaction in front of a crowd of people.

Even when we think we know what's going on it can be hard to plan properly. For example, should the ballplayer take more insulin in anticipation of a BGL spike? What if the game is slow and boring enough that the expected glucose rise doesn't happen? How does the pasta buff know how much insulin resistance the fat content will cause? If you're sick in bed and take insulin in anticipation of a glucose increase from your liver, what happens if you nod off before taking the medicine you planned for?

Here's some practical advice. Don't obsess about occasional high BGLs—they're going to happen. But if we test several times a day we can adjust quickly to fix them. Since the time period between tests is short, planning is easier, too. Instead of trying to guess what your needs will be for an extended amount of time, just plan a few hours ahead and anticipate your need for insulin based on what you know is currently happening. Keeping short accounts with your BGL helps even out lows and highs.

If you like fettucine alfredo, go for it once in a while and control your BGL the best you can based on previous experience. Even if your BGL is high in the morning you can correct it and get back into your routine. If you do this occasionally, it's not a big deal. It's certainly not as traumatic as swearing off your favorite food forever.

Both types of diabetes are complicated and don't always behave the way you think they will. And even if we figure out what works for one person, it may not work that way for another. Each of us is unique and we all have different combinations of activity, food intake, medication, metabolism, organ function and a hundred other things, and they all affect us in different ways. We need professional help to figure this stuff out, and even then it can be puzzling.

If you like riddles, diabetes is the disease for you. Get used to it. Accept the fact that having high BGLs sometimes is part of the game, understand that all diabetics experience them, and then move on without obsessing about it to the point where it robs you of the joy of life.

Chapter 11
Bob Krause

Bob Krause celebrated his 90th birthday in 2011. It was a remarkable milestone because Bob had lived with diabetes for 85 years. He was the first American to do so and he celebrated it at a party where he was presented with a medal from the Joslin Diabetes Center to commemorate his achievement. During his life, he saw diabetic care evolve from sheer hopelessness to realistic management and control. The fact he outlived most non-diabetics his age is astonishing.

Krause was diagnosed in 1926, shortly after insulin became produced commercially and was made widely available. His brother, Jackie, wasn't so fortunate. He had become diabetic a year earlier—too soon to use the new treatment—and died. "I watched Jackie die by starving to death," Krause said. "Before insulin, diabetics would just die because eating doesn't make any difference. Anything that you ate couldn't be converted and you literally starved to death because your body couldn't absorb anything."

His mother wasn't about to lose another child to the disease and when Bob was diagnosed she closely monitored and rigidly limited his food. The idea was to keep his blood sugar as low as possible by reducing the sugars he ingested, which is a good idea even today. Even so, without insulin her strategy would have only marginally prolonged Bob's life while failing to save him from Jackie's fate. But insulin offered real hope and it made young Bob Krause a pioneer in uncharted territory.

Syringes and hypodermic needles were rudimentary. Patients were typically given six needles that would get dull and need to be re-sharpened at home with a whetstone. The glass syringes needed to be boiled between uses. Bob's childhood needles were 25-gauge compared to today's 30-gauge, which means today's are 65% smaller. They had to be big enough to slip a thin wire through to unclog them.

Today they undergo a multi-step sharpening process, are electro-polished to remove painful burrs and are double-lubricated. We're advised not to re-use these ultra-fine modern needles and, if we do, the discomfort is noticeable. It's hard to imagine what it was like to re-use Bob's big old needles after manual sharpening without de-burring or lubrication.

Bob was stuck with this technology and, at the age of six, he injected himself in the legs or arms for each meal. Syringe seals were likely to wear out and affect the accurate measurement of doses, the carbohydrate content of foods was guesswork, and insulin came in different strengths. Mistakenly injecting one strength of insulin at the dosage prescribed for another could be disastrous. Compared to today's knowledge and technology these were truly the dark ages of diabetes management. While insulin enabled his cells to be nourished so he wouldn't starve, accurate control of his BGL was a distant dream. But that problem was small potatoes in the face of one incredible fact...Bob could survive. And that was truly miraculous.

BGL testing was crude. It consisted of boiling urine in a test tube, dropping in a tablet and seeing what color it turned. It measured how much glucose had spilled out of the bloodstream and into the urine an hour or two earlier, so it was a poor indicator of the current BGL. But at least it showed whether you were expelling lots of glucose, which would have indicated that more insulin, less food or both were needed.

Mr. Krause, who died in 2012, owed his success in part to an almost superhuman dedication to restricting his diet. His daily food consumption consisted of prunes and nuts for breakfast, no lunch and then lean meat with salad in the evening. Unless he was going to be physically active—which happened less often as he got older—the regimen didn't change. His mantra was "I eat to live, I don't live to eat."

Bob stuck to his routine throughout his life. His dedication and meticulous control were beyond what most of us are willing or able to do, but Mr. Krause set the gold standard and showed what's possible, even with the primitive technology he used for so many years.

Insulin now comes in a more concentrated standard form, which eliminates the possibility of taking the wrong strength. Since it takes a smaller amount to achieve the same result, we need less insulin and don't beat up injection site tissue as much. In his later years Bob used an insulin pump that only needed to have the infusion site changed once every three days. It was a monumental change for Bob, who still remembered injecting himself with big, dull needles as a child.

My grandparents were born in horse and buggy days and died after astronauts walked on the moon, although my grandmother went to her grave disbelieving the lunar landing. The medical progress Bob Krause saw is at least as amazing.

Speaking of lunar landings, Mr. Krause played a role in getting us there. His career included an engineering professorship at the University of Washington. He left academics after 8 years for the Atlas Rocket Program at General Dynamics where he worked on developing the propulsion technology that put the Mercury astronauts in space. He was later involved in building cruise missiles. That's an impressive resume for anybody, with or without diabetes.

Bob's iron will was no doubt the biggest reason for his health and longevity, but he may also have been blessed with a constitution that tolerated diabetes better than others. Some people have brittle diabetes, which is characterized by frequent, huge swings in the BGL that alternate between very high and extremely low BGLs. It can be brought on by a variety of physical conditions or even psychological factors like stress and depression. It's at the other end of the spectrum from Bob Krause and there are lots of gradations in between.

Here are two examples. One is Casey Johnson, who was diagnosed with Type 1 at age 9 in 1988. She was an heiress to the Johnson & Johnson fortune and had access to the best medical care in the world. Johnson became a party girl and socialite in New York City with an unorthodox but attention-getting lifestyle that culminated in a drug problem. She was 30 when an anonymous 911 caller reported her demise and said Johnson's medications frequently got "all screwed up." She hadn't taken her insulin and died of diabetic ketoacidosis. Her excessive lifestyle produced inattention to diabetes, and it killed her.

The other is Deb Ciosek. She was born into a working class family in the industrial city of Chicopee, MA. One week before her dad was laid off from his factory job and lost their health insurance, Deb was diagnosed with Type 1. She was six years old. For the first twenty years she took just one shot a day with needles that had to be sterilized and re-used, just like Bob Krause. This was ancient technology compared to what Casey Johnson had available, but after over 50 years with diabetes—and good health—she's going strong with no end in sight. Because she's survived so well for so long, the Joslin Diabetes Center has done batteries of tests on her. People who live with diabetes for this long are called "Medalists" by Joslin, and they're literally presented with a medal to commemorate their achievement.

As with other Medalists, the center has invited Deb to donate postmortem tissue samples so they can try to figure out what makes her tick. This isn't a ghoulish exercise and it's not a high-pressure deal. Deb is already a valued participant in the Medalist Study and donations are only accepted from those who have completed it. Participants are told about the organ donation program and that they're welcome to sign up, but if they don't it doesn't affect their status as part of the study.

They've found some surprising things. For example, 100% of the donated pancreases still produced some insulin and many medalists remained free of long-term organ damage. The question is "Why?" The generosity of these donors can give researchers clues to take them in the right, and sometimes unexpected, directions in pursuit of better care and (dare we say it?) a cure.

Different people, different worlds, different approaches to diabetes. One approach is demanding but leads to a successful outcome. The other doesn't. If you have diabetes, the ball is in your court. You can either get in the game like Deb Ciosek and Bob Krause or forfeit it like Casey Johnson. It's your choice.

Chapter 12

Untrue Common "Knowledge"

The common misconceptions about diabetes are enough to drive you crazy. Well-meaning people will do things they think help, but they often don't understand the problem.

Here's a rundown of some common fallacies.

- **Diabetics can't eat sugar.** People often think sugar is toxic for us, but we need glucose for life just like anybody else and can eat sugar as long as our BGL stays reasonable. In fact, when low BGLs happen, sugar is the cure.

- **Diabetes isn't a serious disease.** It kills more people than breast cancer and AIDS put together.

- **Diabetes inevitably leads to amputations and premature death.** With modern diagnostic tools and treatments neither needs to happen as long as the diabetic is attentive to his own daily care.

- **Eating lots of sugar causes diabetes.** Obesity caused by excessive sugar consumption can increase the risk for Type 2 but eating sugar in itself doesn't cause either type.

- **Diabetics need special diets.** A normal, healthy diet for non-diabetic people is also healthy for diabetics. Since the control of blood sugar within a healthy range is important, it's easier to do so if very high sugar foods that will spike the BGL are limited. The bottom line is diabetics can eat anything anybody else does as long as the BGL stays in an acceptable range and they don't gain weight.

- **If a diabetic comes to dinner you'd better watch what you serve.** Well-meaning people sometimes treat us like fine crystal and change the food they offer—usually by reducing sugar content—in order to avoid a "problem" for us. Most of us aren't that fragile, and we can deal with what's in the food. We may choose to avoid problematic foods but nobody needs to change a menu just because a person with diabetes will be at the dinner table.

- **Since fruit is natural and good for you, you can eat as much as you like.** Fruit is a key part of anyone's diet, but they contain carbohydrates that are metabolized into glucose. Because of this they aren't a "free" food that can be consumed without compensating for the carbohydrate content. Sugar is sugar and all sugar, regardless of where it comes from, will raise the BGL.

- **Insulin makes you fat.** Insulin is a hormone that enables your cells to use the glucose in your bloodstream and doesn't make you gain weight by itself.

Just like in non-diabetics, weight gain correlates with food consumption and exercise. If you're sedentary and eat more, your BGL will rise and require more insulin to bring it down. The need for insulin is a consequence of weight-increasing behavior, not the cause of it.

- **You're more likely to get sick than others.** People with diabetes are no more likely to get a cold or the flu than anyone else as long as their BGLs are in good control.

- **Other people can catch the disease from diabetics.** Diabetes is not contagious and can't be spread from person to person.

- **It's preventable and it's your own fault you got it.** When people say it's "preventable" what they really mean (whether they know it or not) is that Type 2 symptoms can be delayed or prevented by keeping weight in check. But both types are caused by triggers that aren't understood and therefore can't be avoided. That being said, researchers believe something in some overweight people does cause insulin resistance although what it is hasn't been definitively identified.

- **All you need to do is take an injection or a pill once a day.** This may be the case with the early stages of Type 2, but otherwise control is an ongoing balancing act that requires adjustments in medical treatment, diet and exercise 24/7/365. Taking oral medications or insulin won't be effective without continual awareness and management.

- **Using insulin causes complications.** People sometimes develop complications from diabetes after starting insulin therapy, but this is the result of waiting too long to start it. The damage is done by previous high BGLs that the insulin will help control.

- **Type 1 diabetes skips generations.** It can appear that way if a grandparent had it, your parent didn't, but then you got it. About 40% of the U.S. population carries the risk gene but only 1% of these get the disease. Your grandparent was one of the unlucky 1% who encountered the trigger but this doesn't indicate greater risk for the grandchildren. However, Type 1 in a parent or sibling *does*.

- **Once you learn how, managing diabetes is easy.** Conditions change continually, even within the course of the day, and it takes constant awareness to make correct adjustments. Diabetics learn routine ways to handle fluctuations but it's not easy, even after you've had the disease for years.

Chapter 13

What If . . . ?

Low sugar reactions need to be identified quickly and treated immediately. Diabetics need to think ahead, judge what their day will be like and plan their strategy. The goal is to keep BGLs low, but not low enough to cause a reaction. But as we all know, sometimes things don't work out as planned and you need be prepared. The question we need to ask is, "What if (fill in the blank) happens?

Nobody's life is the same. Level of activity, mental stress, metabolism, exercise intensity, sensitivity to insulin and lots of other things make us—and our strategies for control—different. But the good news is we can tailor our treatment to our needs. Occupation is a big variable. Secretaries, linebackers, accountants, surgeons, carpenters, coal miners and trapeze artists all place different demands on their bodies and burn off glucose at different rates. Their diabetes strategies vary accordingly.

Life was easier before I got diabetes. I was working to get a new company off the ground. Days were long and packed solid. The operation was a foundry that melted stainless steel and poured it into molds to make industrial castings, so my tasks varied wildly. Sometimes I was doing heavy manual labor, sometimes office work. At times it was brutally hot and at others—particularly on early winter mornings—it could be numbingly cold. Starting any business is stressful, and this was no exception. I ate when I was able to, which sometimes meant not at all.

Diabetes complicated things in a heartbeat. I still needed to do everything I'd always done, but now I had more to think about. Something I never had to consider at all suddenly became my most immediate and constant management problem.

I discovered that hard physical work could drop my BGL to a level that triggered insulin reactions (not a desirable thing while you're pouring molten steel) so I learned to eat more before strenuous work. I kept candy on me so I could eat it if I felt a reaction coming on. This was in the days before blood glucose monitors so I had to rely on my symptoms to tell me if the BGL was going low.

It could be a dicey situation because some of them, like sweating and feeling slightly weak, could be confused with what happens when you're working hard physically. The rule was "if you're not sure, treat for low blood sugar" so I'd eat some carbs, continue working and check the urine for spilled sugar later. This would tell me whether I guessed right or wrong.

Dealing with diabetes affected my life in very practical ways but I managed to work around them. Like we all do. Each of us has different circumstances to contend with, some more demanding than others. Here are a few:

Charlie Kimball is a racecar driver who speeds around the track at 190 mph in a job that requires lightning-fast reflexes. He's also got Type 1, the only person with the disease cleared to race professionally. Charlie's job requires intense effort for long periods and mental acuity is critical. High or low BGLs will affect this, so extraordinarily tight control is required.

He monitors his BGL just like he checks his car's oil pressure and temperature—by checking a digital readout. Kimball wears a continuous glucose monitor that checks his BGL and radios it to a screen mounted on his steering wheel. If the BGL drops too much the driver is prepared with an old-school solution—he drinks orange juice from a straw installed in his helmet. For Charlie Kimball, it's just another indicator he's got to keep track of. Charlie's question is "What if I'm doing 195 mph and my BGL drops?"

The Chicago Cubs were/are chronically inept. It's part of their charm. But Ron Santo, a 13-year Cubs third baseman, was a winner who was inducted into the Baseball Hall of Fame. Santo had Type 1 diabetes when he came up from the minors and believed his career would be jeopardized if the team found out about it, so he kept it to himself. It was the early 1960's and he may have been right about that.

Blood glucose monitors wouldn't be widely available for decades, so Santo had to diagnose low sugar the old fashioned way—be aware of sweating, blurry vision, weakness and mood changes—and then eat sugar before he lost his mental acuity.

He once was on-deck on a sweltering afternoon. Hot weather complicates things because you're sweating anyway, and it's sometimes hard to know if it's from the heat or a low BGL. The Cubs were down 2-0 with two men out and two on base in the bottom of the 9th. Suddenly an insulin reaction sneaked up on him. He became woozy and hoped the batter at the plate would make an out to end the game and let him get to the dugout for a candy bar. The furthest thing from his mind was going back to the dugout and explaining why he was there to hard-as-nails Manager Leo Durocher.

But the batter walked, loading the bases and bringing Santo to the plate amid the screams of 20,000 fans. Seeing in triple, he looked up to see three pitchers winding up and throwing a pitch that came in "looking like it was attached to a Slinky." Ron swung at it and put the ball out of the park for a walk-off grand slam home run.

It's a great story, but look at the "what if's." What if a manager called a time out? Or the pitcher threw balls? Or Santo fouled some pitches off? Or the umpire decided to check the ball or sweep the plate? A little more time without sugar and he could have collapsed into an incoherent heap.

In fairness, Ron Santo was a gutsy guy in a bad situation who didn't have the tools to know his predicament until it was too late. Today a player can be open about diabetes without fear of being fired and can know his BGL before going on deck. No doubt Santo would have loved to have had those advantages. Ron's question was, "What if I have a reaction when I'm in a game?"

Life is fraught with "What if's." What if…

You go for a boat ride that lasts a lot longer than you thought it would? Bring more carbs than you think you'll need. Unless the boat has a snack bar or soda machine you're on your own to avoid a low BGL.

Your plane gets held up for hours on the tarmac? Tell a flight attendant you have diabetes so they'll understand the urgency if you ask for sugar, sugar soda or high-carb foods.

An accident turns the highway into a parking lot? Think of your vehicle as a Conestoga wagon that carries everything you need. It should always have foods that won't spoil, like breakfast bars. Glucose tablets are compact and you can fit lots of them in a glove compartment.

You get stuck in a long meeting and can't eat when you planned? Casually eat some candy or glucose tablets, or get yourself a sugared drink. If you don't want to be conspicuous you don't need to be.

You go on a "hike" that was supposed to last two hours but turned out to be four hours of steep climbing?

This actually happened to me. Bring a backpack with more fruit bars and glucose tablets than you think you could possibly need. They're high-carb, light and compact. If you still run short be sure your companions know what's going on.

I once took a boat for what should have been a quick ride across the lake to the mechanic's dock, but it died halfway there. I had been in a hurry and jumped in with only the candy in my pocket. Suddenly I found myself alone with the possibility of having to paddle the rest of the way. This would have dropped my BGL and I wasn't confident I had enough sugar on me to avoid a reaction.

It was a classic "How could I be so stupid?" moment. Luckily I managed to get the attention of another boat that towed me in. Everything turned out OK, but it might not have. Things like this are the reason we need to think ahead...always. Minor inconveniences can turn into dangerous situations very quickly if you're unprepared.

You get the idea. Situations where low sugar reactions can occur crop up all over the place, and putting thought into even the most common activities is a routine part of living with diabetes.

Chapter 14

Unsung Heroes

Diabetes presents a whole bunch of problems for those who live with diabetics. It's serious business, and you'd have to be in a discussion group with people who live with diabetics to understand how universal the difficulties they face are. They're patient, understanding, loving, supportive, frustrated, exasperated and sometimes angry—occasionally all at the same time. They are unsung heroes.

We diabetics are chained to this disease, but so are our spouses and families. We take the medications, count the carbs, adjust our lifestyles, endure the highs and lows, and do our best to manage it. It's a steady drumbeat of decision making and there's no break from it. And all the while our unsung heroes sit on the sidelines hoping for the best but knowing a low blood sugar reaction could be right around the corner.

Managing diabetes wears on you. You're doing your best—but often failing to meet your own expectations—and you don't really want to hear advice or criticism from anybody else. Especially somebody who doesn't have diabetes and can't possibly know what it's like to be in your shoes. It's probably one reason we can be stubborn.

It's said we can be irritable, sometimes in a way that implies we're resentful cusses with bad attitudes. The truth is even temporary high BGLs can make you tired, drowsy and annoyed with yourself because you've got lots to do and just don't feel up to it. On the other hand, low BGLs can dull your mental sharpness and force you to drop what you're doing to eat sugar. Irritability isn't something we deliberately foist on others. It's got physiological roots and is something we work to overcome, but it can make us hard to live with. Considering that everybody—diabetic or not—can be hard to live with anyway, I guess we're in a class of our own.

Unsung heroes come in lots of packages. When Ron Santo (the diabetic baseball Hall of Famer who kept his condition secret) finally confided to his roommate, it turned out to be a great thing. Sometimes when Santo came off the field his friend would say, "Roomie, you look a little pale. Better grab a Snickers."

My wife does the same thing, except she doesn't call me "roomie." She knows the tip-offs—a sweat-soaked bed sheet is an obvious one, but sometimes she puts her hand on me when I'm sleeping and can tell if I'm having a reaction by the texture of my skin. The indicators vary by individual and are usually subtle—the kind of thing only someone very close to you would notice. Things like slight slowness of speech, delayed responses to questions, changes in the way you walk or move, odd laughter or a hundred other things. They vary among individuals and may change over time.

It took me a long time to stop resenting my wife when she asked, "do you need something to eat?" because I prided myself on being self-sufficient. I was the one actually living in this body and believed I knew best. Except sometimes I didn't and would find myself having the insulin reaction my wife already told me was coming. Part of the problem is when your BGL is too low you lose your ability to think clearly, which is why it's important to listen to your unsung hero.

My wife isn't always right. She can be fooled when I'm sweating because I'm hot but not having a reaction, for example. Here's the strategy: when she speaks, I listen. If my blood glucose meter is close by, I do a test. If it isn't, I ask myself how I feel, what I've been doing, how long it's been since I ate and what my last BGL was. If this adds up to the BGL possibly being low, I eat something sugary. If I'm not sure, I still eat something sugary. Even if I guess wrong and the BGL isn't low, a temporary high BGL is small price to pay to avoid a possibly bad reaction.

Sometimes unsung heroes deal with someone whose BGL has gone low enough to make his brain to go haywire. Unlike other cells in the body, brain cells don't store glucose. When the BGL plummets these cells are immediately starved and can't function, which means you can't think. It's not like taking a sedative or diet pill that can cause you to think slower or faster but still keep your thought processes orderly. There's no point in trying to reason with someone having a reaction because they literally can't be logical. In my case, random disorganized thoughts flit into my mind and disappear as quickly as they came. They can be from past experiences or involve current things I'm worried about, and they tend to be negative. They pop into my head with increasing speed and frequency and the lower the BGL goes, the worse it gets. Caleb, the little boy with Type 1 discussed in Chapter 4, once recovered from a reaction and told his mom he thought he was a crab. You'd have to experience this to know how bizarre the circus in your head can become.

There's a point of no return. If you're lucid enough to know you're having a reaction you can eat sugar to raise your BGL. But if you don't treat it in time, your brain becomes foggy and even though your symptoms are getting bad your weakened brain cells won't let you recognize it. If you don't get help at this point you'll lose consciousness.

What's an unsung hero to do when this happens? First, they can try to get you to drink something sugary—like orange juice mixed with sugar. If that doesn't work and you pass out, they can inject you with glucagon or call the EMT's. However they handle it, your unsung hero is thrown into an adrenaline-pumping emergency.

And you? Once the BGL is back up you recover and don't remember much, if anything, about the drama. You're exhausted and will go right to sleep, but your unsung hero won't nod off so easily. Severely low BGLs like this should be rare, but our unsung heroes know the drill when they do occur.

They're always on the lookout to prevent them from happening. When they see the symptoms they understandably want to decisively raise the BGL with lots of sugar, but it's easy to overshoot the need and send the sugar level way too high. Here's a tip. If the diabetic is lucid it means his brain cells are on line. Have him check his BGL. If he can't do it himself, he's probably still got a very low BGL and you should insist he eat some sugar. But if he can do his own test, hold off on blasting him with sugar and make adjustments based on his actual BGL.

Living with someone who has diabetes isn't easy. Those who do are unsung heroes who deserve love, thanks, respect and praise.

Chapter 15

Dear Friends and Relatives:
A Chapter to Share with Others

You probably don't know much about diabetes, and that's understandable. I didn't either until I got it. Like most of you, I knew people who had diabetes and they seemed to be doing OK, so I figured it couldn't be very big deal. Boy, was I wrong. As a retired friend who was recently diagnosed said, "This is really nasty."

Let me explain. Diabetes causes high levels of sugar (also called glucose) in the bloodstream and this can cause major health problems. While a non-diabetic body automatically controls the blood glucose level (called BGL for short), diabetic ones don't. Diabetics need to control the BGL artificially by taking insulin and/or medications. These keep us from dying, which was what happened before treatments were available.

Lots of factors determine my BGL. Sugars and starches raise it. Coffee raises it. Insulin reduces it. Medications can reduce it. Exercise reduces it. With all these ways to reduce it, you'd think it would be easy to keep it really low, and it could be. Except there's a problem—if the BGL goes too low it can disrupt my ability to think straight and affect coordination. If it gets extremely low I could pass out.

The need to keep the BGL from being too high or too low is what makes this complicated. Diabetics can't just take a pill or injection once a day and then forget about it because the things we do during the day change the BGL. We have to adjust to activities, medications, what we've eaten, and other things. We constantly try to maintain balance, but it can be elusive.

What we eat is important. We try to determine how many carbohydrates we're consuming because these become glucose when they're digested and that's what causes our BGLs to rise. We know the carb content of foods we commonly eat, but in some situations we don't know them and need to make educated guesses. Think about it. How many carbs are in Aunt Sally's secret recipe for three-bean salad, the local pizza joint's marinara sauce or picnics where everybody brings something? Fortunately, after you've dealt with this for a time you develop a good enough idea of carb contents to be able to guess them adequately.

Once we know this we can compensate for it. For example, we can adjust our portions, take insulin, or burn it off with exercise afterward.

Occasionally falling off the tight balance wagon won't kill us; in fact having temporary high or low BGLs is unavoidable. Getting back in control is the important thing because there are serious consequences for having chronically high BGLs.

We're living on a tightrope trying to keep our balance between too high and too low and it isn't easy. It's even more daunting because there's never a break from it—awake, asleep, working, exercising, tossing a ball, watching a show… it's always there.

Most of us know what we're doing, so it's annoying to have a non-diabetic give you a jaundiced eye when you take a piece of pie, a scoop of ice cream or—God forbid—pie a la mode! I assume they do this because they think sugar is poison to us and we're behaving recklessly.

But sugar in itself isn't the problem—it's whether our BGL is in balance (meaning in a target range that's not too high or too low). In fact, if the BGL is too low, we need to eat sugar to raise it up to the target range. If a diabetic knows the carb content of a dessert and takes enough insulin to cover the sugar he's eating, he'll keep his BGL in control just like your body automatically does for you. Diabetics try to mimic the natural mechanism by taking the correct dosage of insulin for the amount of food ingested.

Unsurprisingly, most non-diabetics don't understand this. But some people feel free to judge a diabetic's food consumption based on their own misconceptions. This phenomenon is so common and annoying that the diabetes community calls them the "diabetes police." Articles offer advice on handling them, especially around the holidays when you're bound to eat something sugary in public.

Sometimes the police are silent – but their eyes speak volumes and the diabetic figures gossip will be circulating soon. Other times, they'll ask if you should "really be eating that." There are four possible responses. First, you could not eat the food—but this just empowers the questioner. ("Put the doughnut down now and nobody gets hurt!") Second, tell them "It's no problem: I've got it under control." That will work, but you'll probably be rewarded with a skeptical look. Third, give an impromptu diabetes lesson that will interrupt conversation and may sound rude. Finally, you can tell them you're OK and if they would like to know more, you can set up a time to talk about it later.

There are no quick, effective answers. But it would sure help if the diabetes police just read this chapter.

This isn't to imply you should never bring diabetes up. One helpful thing is to ask if we'd like to know how many carbs are in the dishes you're serving. The information is usually on food packaging. If you don't know, don't sweat it. We're pretty good at estimating carbs and, if we're uncertain, we'll take small portions of questionable foods or none at all. And please know this: if my BGL gets temporarily high I might get a little sluggish (like we all do after a big Thanksgiving dinner) but it won't be a dangerous "Call 911" situation.

Low BGLs are different. There are serious, immediate consequences to an untreated low BGL, and these may well require EMT's if they're not treated in time. If you remember anything from this chapter, please make it this: if a diabetic tells you he's got to eat, it's not because he's got a sudden hankering for food. It's because he knows his BGL is getting low and he's got to eat some carbohydrate/sugar to avoid a reaction. If he needs to eat, let him do it without a hassle.

If you've spent time with a diabetic you've no doubt been there when his BGL has been low, even if you didn't know it. This isn't an unusual occurrence, especially if a person is trying to maintain tight control. Low BGLs may be a sign the person is seriously working to avoid chronically high blood sugars. But those who don't understand may roll their eyes because "Uncle Bob's sugar is low again" when he may actually deserve credit.

Indications that the BGL is too low can include sweating, slowness of speech, loss of mental acuity, impaired coordination and others. Low BGLs require sugar to raise them and easily digestible high sugar foods will do the trick. Sugar mixed in orange juice works well but other high sugar sources will also do the job. If a person isn't responding or can't eat, don't force feed him because he may choke. At this point, you should call the EMT's. It's a routine thing for them and they'll take care of it quickly.

Having said all this, the chances are you'll never have to deal with it. Most of us are well aware of our situation and deal with highs and lows smoothly enough that you don't even know we're doing it.

We can't afford to tire of dealing with diabetes, but it's nice to forget about it for a little while. Many of us keep our condition to ourselves and only share it with certain people, just as others keep their ailments private.

If you have a diabetic over you could help with this. Carbohydrate information is appreciated if you have it, but please offer it privately. I've been to dinners where somebody announced they reduced the sugar in this or that because I've got diabetes. It makes me wince because the information isn't useful without knowing the carb content and – worse – it makes diabetes the table topic.

This can be uncomfortable because there's often a sense of misplaced pity that many diabetics neither need nor want. On top of this, like lots of other people, many of us prefer to stay on the sidelines and aren't comfortable being the center of attention for any reason, especially diabetes.

For most of my years with diabetes I didn't talk about it with people I didn't know well for one reason. The word "diabetic" can conjure up an incorrect stereotype of who I am. I'm not frail, sickly or needy and I pursue life as actively and competently as anyone else. Diabetes doesn't establish my identity any more than blindness defines Stevie Wonder. And like other diabetics, I deal with it well enough that people don't know I have it unless I tell them. To be honest, broadcasting the fact I have diabetes is the hardest thing about writing this book.

It's hard to fault people for having incorrect ideas. After all, they only know what they see. It could be that a relative became blind, got into a car accident or died young because of it. Years ago serious complications were largely unavoidable. Fortunately, today many of them can be dealt with effectively.

But they still happen when diabetics don't manage their disease. A guy who worked for me years ago totally ignored his Type 2 and finally went to the hospital with necrosis in 2012.

Surgeons amputated both his legs, one on one day and the other on the next. It doesn't take many stories like this to leave the impression that diabetics hopelessly come to bad ends. But what they really show is that if you don't take care of yourself the disease is as devastating as ever.

Sometimes people think diabetes is something we brought on ourselves by, for example, eating too much sugar or that we could cure ourselves if we just lost some weight. Here are some facts.

There are two primary types of diabetes, aptly named Type 1 and Type 2. Science doesn't know how either originates, but it does know a lot. Type 1 is caused by the immune system killing the body's insulin producing cells. Type 2 is caused by the inability of the body's cells to use insulin in a condition called insulin resistance. While there's a connection between obesity and Type 2, it's vexing because thin people also get it while many overweight people don't. Both types result in cells starving and excess sugar floating in the blood.

Weight loss won't rejuvenate a Type 1 pancreas or eliminate insulin resistance. But controlling weight is important to managing both types.

Uninformed non-diabetics tend to be in one of three camps. The "Poor Soul" people think you can't eat sugar—so desserts are dangerous—and that you're always on the edge of some vague disaster, so it makes sense to keep half and eye on you. The "Get Over It" crowd knows it's something we need to deal with, although they don't know why or how, but the disease is so common it can't be a big deal. The "No Problem" faction thinks diabetes is easily controlled with medication and it's no more involved than toe fungus.

They're all wrong. The "Poor Soul" people should know sugar isn't a poison but something diabetics need. The "Get Over It" group should realize that more people die from diabetes than breast cancer and AIDS combined. And "No Problem" people should know this is a relentless 24/7/365 deal that requires constant vigilance. Let me go out on a limb and speak for all diabetics everywhere: We would trade diabetes for toe fungus any day of the week and twice on Sundays.

Thanks for reading this. There's an epidemic of diabetes and we all need to know what's going on. You now know more about it than most people, and all of us who grapple with it appreciate your willingness to understand it better.

And please do a big favor for yourself and everyone who loves you. Get yourself screened for diabetes. It's quick and easy but it could be one of the most important things you ever do.

Chapter 16

Occupational Considerations

Some jobs used to be off-limits to diabetics mainly because of possible low sugar reactions. Here's an example of this thinking:

> "Firemen are rousted out of bed in the middle of the night, rush to put on gear, jump on a truck, race to a fire, hook up heavy hoses to hydrants, and climb ladders to smash holes in roofs. There's no time for a BGL check or even eating something in the rush, and once on site the work is strenuous, stressful, and non-stop. Firemen can instantly find themselves in life-saving or life-threatening situations, neither of which is a good place for a low sugar reaction. Allowing diabetics to be firemen is just not worth the risk."

The American Diabetes Association (ADA) has worked to open up all sorts of jobs to diabetics, including firefighting and law enforcement. As a result diabetes can't legally be used as an automatic disqualification for employment; applicants must be assessed individually on whether they can safely and effectively function in the jobs. You might think this is an impossibly high bar to clear, but diabetics got these jobs and proved they could perform them as well as anybody else. These trailblazers taught us how and why they've been successful.

Some of the practical things they do include keeping high sugar drinks in the fire truck, making sure glucose tablets are always in their gear, and taking insulin after they eat just in case an alarm comes in during a meal. Perhaps surprisingly, low BGLs during heavy action haven't turned out to be a problem.

When humans find themselves in "fight or flight" situations—like fighting a fire—the body releases adrenaline. This prompts the liver to release the glucose the body needs for energy to respond to the stressful situation.

This happens in both Type 1 and Type 2 firefighters and it's a reason they can perform these jobs without going low. One firefighter put it this way, "I rarely get low during a call or fire as my firefighting instinct takes over and I just do my job. The lows strike when everything calms down and then my body decides: 'Hey, you just burned a lot of (carbohydrates) and you didn't replace them.'"* In other words, the adrenaline prompted the liver to pump glucose into the bloodstream for as long as it was needed, which prevented a low BGL. But after the action was over, the liver's stored glucose was depleted and the firefighter needed to eat. It's not necessarily an immediate thing—sometimes they don't need to eat right away because the lows can happen hours after the event. Insulin dependent diabetics have demonstrated a counterintuitive fact—they perform under physical and mental pressure as well as anyone else without risking low BGLs.

Law enforcement officers are in essentially the same position as firefighters. There are many of them doing great jobs and they, too, have dismantled barriers for diabetics because of their proven performance.

---

*Ginger Vieira, Fighting Fires with Type 1 Diabetes, 9/7/2012, *www.diabetesdaily.com*

Despite these successes there are some occupations that are restricted in one way or another. They include:

Commercial Driving

Diabetics can be granted an exemption from USDOT medical requirements and allowed to drive in interstate commerce. You'll need to be screened by a medical examiner, present logs, pass a visual exam conducted by an ophthalmologist or optometrist and meet other requirements. If an exemption is granted you're required to submit quarterly and annual medical and monitoring reports, have medical re-certification exams annually and reapply to renew the exemption every two years. There a lot of hoops to jump through but at least there's a realistic chance to get a Commercial Driver's License.

Military Service

Both types disqualify diabetics from enlistment. If a person is diagnosed with Type 1 or Type 2 while in the service, an involved medical review procedure is followed and a discharge may or may not be issued depending upon the severity, level of control and position held. Those with administrative positions are less likely to be discharged than combatants. It can take persistence to fight the system, but there are cases where diabetics with both types have been allowed to stay in the military.

Some occupations have restrictions for persons with diabetes. But in the grand scheme of things, how many areas are truly off-limits? Not the butcher, the baker or the candlestick maker. Or doctors, nurses, computer geeks, farmers, manufacturing workers, cooks, mechanics, salespeople, executives, construction workers, teachers, artists, engineers or most of the other jobs on this planet.

Employers aren't legally allowed to ask medical questions before an applicant is hired, so diabetics can apply for jobs and get hired on their merits. Once the job is offered, employers can require a medical exam but can only refuse to hire you if a medical workup indicates your diabetes will impair your ability to perform the job in question. But employers aren't required to do this and it may not be an issue for you at all.

If the question does arise, it's best to seek the advice of a diabetes professional to provide an individual assessment. If the employer's physician doesn't have expertise in this area (and many don't) you can provide an individualized assessment from one who knows you, like your own doctor. A physician who is familiar with your history and the control you've demonstrated over time will have the most credibility. And as a bonus, medical people often have personal relationships with their patients and want them to do well. They may be more objective than a "doc for hire" who may be inclined to say "no" just because he's not sure and wants to avoid legal liability.

Employers aren't necessarily the bad guys. They have responsibilities to their customers and other employees, and they may have a legal liability if they knowingly hire someone who can't perform due to a medical condition. On one hand they can understandably be cautious. On the other hand, they're always looking for good people and any employer worth his salt would happily hire a qualified diabetic candidate who received a thumbs-up from a physician.

Thanks to the work of the ADA and others, many previously closed doors have swung open and the range of opportunities for diabetics has become wider than ever.

Chapter 17

Working on a Cure

Sometimes it seems like progress is being made in curing every disease but this one. Just to keep us on our toes, every so often the press breathlessly teases us with a "breakthrough" that turns out to be hype. So far, none of the magical mystery cures has held up.

In fairness to the scientists who really are working tirelessly on this, both types of diabetes are complicated diseases that expose unknown wrinkles as new research paths are followed. On top of their intrinsic difficulties, Type 1 and Type 2 present radically different problems and because they're so dissimilar, research on one often doesn't apply to the other. Funding for research is divided between them.

Let's talk about Type 1 first. Science still doesn't know why it happens, but it's clearly an autoimmune disease in which the diabetic's own antibodies treat insulin-producing cells as foreign intruders and kills them. This autoimmune response is always present and it becomes progressively more lethal the longer a person has the disease. Any new cells implanted into a Type 1 person need to somehow counter this or be killed off just like the original cells.

It's a vexing problem.

It's possible to suppress the general immune system to allow beta cells to survive, but the cure is worse than the disease. A compromised immune system makes the body vulnerable to all sorts of invaders. With no defense against microscopic threats, death from non-diabetic causes would be more likely than from diabetes, so it is currently a "pick your poison" proposition. Choosing to deal with diabetes over some other disease your weakened system could enable may be wise.

Researchers have identified the specific autoimmune cells that attack the beta cells. They're called "T cells" and vaccines that specifically suppress them have cured diabetes in mice. But so far long term success in humans hasn't panned out.

In one successful human experiment, researchers extracted the cells that are precursors to immune system cells. Then they used drugs to kill off the subject's immune system and reintroduced the previously harvested cells, which hadn't been affected by the trigger that turned the old cells into beta cell attackers. Most of the test subjects were still producing insulin over two years after the procedure was performed. So far the side effects appear to be minor and it seems to be the only current treatment potentially capable of reversing Type 1.

Reconstructing the immune system is only part of the solution because the body still needs to have functioning beta cells and these have largely been killed off. There are several approaches to this. One is to grow new cells outside the body and then transplant them. Another could use drugs to coax existing live cells into producing new ones that haven't been compromised by the deadly T cells. They can also be supplied by the pancreases of deceased organ donors, and work is being done to enable the use of animal sources, like pig pancreases. This isn't a big stretch because porcine insulin was used in humans for many years until we learned to synthesize human insulin.

Work is being done on the implantation of a membrane containing beta cells. The idea is to develop a fabric porous enough to let glucose in and insulin out, but fine enough to exclude T cells. Scientists cured diabetic rats this way in 1980, but human application has been slowed by problems in developing a workable membrane material, determining the best location for implants and finding the best cell types to use.

While a biological cure is proving elusive, other scientists are developing an artificial pancreas that would mimic the operation of the real thing. Versions have already been made that combine the existing technologies of the continuous glucose meter, insulin pump and a computer that calculates the dosage. It has the potential for revolutionizing treatment by tightly controlling the BGL and removing the threat of low blood sugar. The ultimate goal is to build an implantable device that could truly take over the constant management decisions we make now. It wouldn't be a cure, but it would sure feel like one.

In the meantime, research at the Joslin Medalist Study aims to prevent or reverse complications. Although these aren't cures they hope to decrease rates of eye problems and potentially fatal kidney disease. The study is also trying to "turn on" the insulin-producing beta cells found to exist in pancreases otherwise compromised by Type 1.

Type 2 is different. A cure would need to solve two problems—inadequate insulin production and insulin resistance. Researchers are looking at ways to regenerate damaged cells in the pancreas, which would help restore natural production. This may work more readily in Type 2 because it's not an autoimmune disease like Type 1 and the newly functioning beta cells wouldn't be killed off by renegade T cells. But it wouldn't solve the insulin resistance problem, which is not well understood and is probably the more difficult condition to address. Until scientists learn more about insulin resistance a cure is probably not imminent.

There is an intriguing development, though. Bariatric surgery reconfigures the stomach and other parts of the digestive system to limit how much can be eaten, reduce the amount of nutrients that can be absorbed by the body, or both. It's a weight loss procedure that's sometimes performed on Type 2 diabetics who haven't been able to drop weight through diet and exercise. A side effect of the surgery is the remission of Type 2—even before weight loss occurs. Nobody knows why this happens, but a theory is that hormonal changes are triggered when the digestive tract is reconfigured. However this happens, the body regains its ability to use insulin and process glucose. Like so many other medical breakthroughs, the clue was stumbled upon, and researchers are actively pursuing it.

A study was done comparing a control group that had no surgery to two others that underwent two different bariatric procedures. The control group saw no remission of diabetes, but one surgery produced a 95% remission rate and the other 75%. While the surgery isn't currently recommended for non-obese patients some researchers see it being used for this in the future.

With both types of diabetes there is ongoing research and someday researchers will solve the puzzles. You never know—scientists are toiling as we speak and might be on the cusp of truly earth shaking cures.

In the meantime, others are developing even better equipment and therapies to help us survive in good health. Even without cures, technological advances in managing diabetes have revolutionized the ease and effectiveness of treatment and will continue to give us even better lives in the future.

Chapter 18
Will Cross

Climbing Mount Everest is a staggering challenge. Strength, endurance and mental toughness are required on a mountain that drains climbers of all of them.

Extreme cold is a real danger. Storms can spring up suddenly with hurricane force winds, whipping the snow so densely you sometimes can't see your feet. You can't see well enough to find shelter and can't blindly grope for it because a wrong step could send you falling thousands of feet. The best bet can be huddling in place and hoping the storm blows over before you freeze.

Low body temperature is called hypothermia and its effects are serious. They start with shivering and mental confusion, progress into loss of coordination, stumbling and impaired circulation, then move into irrational or incoherent behavior. Paradoxical undressing can occur, which is a phenomenon in which severely hypothermic victims remove their clothing. But as bad as this can be, the cold isn't the biggest threat.

That distinction goes to hypoxia, or oxygen deprivation. The air is so thin at Everest's altitudes that a climber needs to take three breaths to take in as much oxygen as one breath at sea level. It wreaks havoc with the digestive system, which needs lots of oxygen to metabolize food. Climbers can experience a loss of appetite and gastrointestinal distress. Even worse, it affects mental sharpness. Climbers have said they feel dizzy, drugged, delirious and disengaged as their cognitive functions diminish. Some have blackouts or hallucinations. Jon Krakauer, an Everest summiteer and author of the book *Into Thin Air*, recalls being in a "state of hypoxic imbecility." All this in a place where turning the wrong way can cost you your life.

The cold, oxygen deficient stretch between 25,000 feet and the summit at 29,035 is called the "Death Zone" because it has earned the name. Expeditions require climbers to sign waivers acknowledging that if they die on the mountain their bodies will be left behind. It's estimated that over 200 remain, some down in crevasses or buried in snow, others in view at the spots where they died. "Green Boots" is the nickname given to the deceased climber who still wears them. His frozen body has been there since 1996 and is now a landmark on the way up.

Imagine trying this with diabetes. You'd be up there facing major league physical distress compounded by your disease. Even though your body would need to burn carbohydrates by the boatload you may have a lack of appetite and an impaired ability to digest food. This could dramatically and unpredictably affect your treatment regimen. And adding the possibility of a low sugar reaction to a brain already stressed by hypothermia and hypoxia would seem practically suicidal. If there's a place diabetics should avoid, this would be it.

But Will Cross didn't see it that way. Cross was diagnosed with Type 1 when he was nine years old, but it was just a speed bump for an adventurous spirit. With proper training and control he trekked to the North and South Poles on foot and climbed six of the Seven Summits (the highest peaks on each of the continents). Then he conquered Everest, the seventh summit.

How did he do it? For starters, he kept his insulin near his body so it wouldn't freeze. It was always in his climbing suit or in his sleeping bag. Upon rising at 3:00AM, Will checked his BGL and again several hours after eating and suiting up. After the day's climbing he checked again and then one final time before turning in.

To meet the need for digestible carbs he consumed sports gels and energy bars about every hour. Since testing was impractical outside the protection of a tent, Will monitored his BGL the old fashioned way, by paying close attention to his body's signals and relying on the predictability of his insulin. He also educated his teammates on the symptoms and treatment of a low BGL.

Cross used an insulin pump on the ascent but was concerned the very low ambient air pressure might disable it. He brought flexpens along so he could inject the insulin if the pump went down, but it didn't. The pump worked fine and now he plans to use a continuous glucose monitoring device on his next climb. This should help remove uncertainty about his BGL that could arise due to the symptomatic similarities between a low BGL and hypoxia.

He's a man with a mission who says, "I hope this sends a clear message to people living with diabetes that if they carefully control their disease, they can attempt to tackle anything." Will has Type 1 diabetes and an unbeatable can-do spirit. He said, "I only had two choices with this thing—one was to whine about it and one was to do something about it."

It's hard to explain diabetes without giving the impression diabetics are constantly on the edge of disaster and shouldn't push the envelope. But if you control it – and refuse to let it control you – anything is possible. Just ask Will Cross.

Afterword

If you have diabetes you may feel that living with it and controlling it is complicated and hard to do. You'd be right about that.

You may also feel you're trapped on a runaway train to bad health, disastrous complications and a shortened life. Whether that's true or not depends largely on you and your ability to control your BGLs. It's a huge responsibility that rests squarely on your shoulders.

Diabetes adds an exasperating complexity to life. But we need to accept we're stuck with it, play the cards we're dealt and know we'll do fine if we play them skillfully.

Chapter 3 listed some highly successful people with diabetes. They're living on a tightrope just like you and have overcome the challenges of diabetes to excel at what they do. The rest of us may not be famous but, like them, we wrestle with the beast every day to live productive, satisfying, healthy and long lives. With a smile.

If this sounds like you, give yourself a pat on the back. You deserve it!

About the Author

C. William "Chet" Galaska began his college education at Drew University in Madison, NJ and graduated from the University of Hartford, West Hartford, CT with a Bachelor's Degree in Business Administration. He was president and co-founder of a company producing stainless steel and high alloy castings for industrial applications. In 2003, he sold his interest in the operation and now writes and invests in real estate.

He's not a medical person, but is someone who has had Type 1 diabetes since 1981. He offers a practical look at this disease from a patient's point of view and explains a number of things diabetics often learn the hard way.

He played rugby, earned a Private Pilot's License, is a Certified Scuba Diver, has skydived, likes roller coasters and enjoys traveling.

He and his wife Lisa live in Western Massachusetts.

Made in the USA
Lexington, KY
13 May 2015